LIVING YOUR HEALTHIEST SEMAGLUTIDE LIFE

DEDICATION

For those who have struggled, felt hopeless, or once believed that losing weight was impossible: This book is for you. To the ones who've felt weighed down by more than just physical challenges, who've faced judgment, self-doubt, and the exhaustion of trying over and over again, doing all the things—I see you. Please know we are just at the very beginning of this new age of obesity care. This book is dedicated to those of us who have struggled long enough.

Quarto.com

© 2025 Quarto Publishing Group USA Inc.
Text © 2025 Summer Kessel

First Published in 2025 by Fair Winds Press,
an imprint of The Quarto Group, 100 Cummings Center, Suite 265-D, Beverly, MA 01915, USA.
T (978) 282-9590 F (978) 283-2742

Fair Winds Press titles are also available at discount for retail, wholesale, promotional, and bulk purchase. For details, contact the Special Sales Manager by email at specialsales@quarto.com or by mail at The Quarto Group, Attn: Special Sales Manager, 100 Cummings Center, Suite 265-D, Beverly, MA 01915, USA.

29 28 27 26 25   1 2 3 4 5

ISBN: 978-0-7603-9616-2

Digital edition published in 2025
eISBN: 978-0-7603-9617-9

Library of Congress Cataloging-in-Publication Data available

Design, Page Layout, and Illustration: Emily Austin, The Sly Studio

Printed in China

The information in this book is for educational purposes only. It is not intended to replace the advice of a physician or medical practitioner. Please see your health care provider before beginning any new health program.

LIVING YOUR

A COMPLETE GUIDE TO **NUTRITION**

HEALTHIEST

AND **MINDSET** WHILE ON GLP-1 MEDICATIONS

SEMAGLUTIDE LIFE

SUMMER KESSEL, RD, CSOWM, LDN

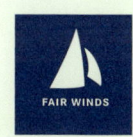

FAIR WINDS

CONTENTS

FOREWORD

by Dr. Spencer Nadolsky, Obesity and Lipid Specialist Physician

When I first met Summer, it was actually via an X (formerly Twitter) chat about nutrition. She later joined the obesity telemedicine service I created to get access to a GLP-1 medicine for help with her weight. I was looking for new dietitians to join the program to help our patients. She was so excited to help other people going through what she was going through that she even accepted a pay cut compared to what she was making as a dietitian in the hospital.

It was very clear that Summer cared passionately for her clients. She learned everything there was to learn about these medicines while also developing nutritional strategies for patients that would minimize side effects and keep them engaged in the program. And with all that, she would also jump in and help in terms of customer service issues if a patient had fallen through the cracks for one reason or another.

Summer exemplifies how obesity and weight struggles go far beyond knowledge of nutrition and exercise and discipline. She is an extremely knowledgeable dietitian with an impeccable work ethic; even still, she struggled with her weight before using a GLP-1 medicine. Because of this experience, she is very relatable to other people going through the same journey. She understands the stigma patients face and the hardships they go through when trying to lose weight and keep it off.

This book is an extension of her that combines her wealth of knowledge, not only about nutrition and exercise but also about her journey.

PREFACE

If you know me at all, as some of you do from our years together on social media, I'm so thankful you are here. If you don't know me, my name is Summer, and I'm a registered dietitian nutritionist who has finally found my niche in the management of nutrition for people on GLP-1 medication. I'm also a late-thirtysomething mom of two who has struggled with my weight my entire life—I have the chronic disease of obesity—who finally found my personal solution with the assistance of GLP-1 medication. I'm beyond grateful to have written this book for you as a guide on your journey with GLP-1 treatment. It will be vulnerable and transparent and, hopefully, relatable. Let's be real, this is scary.

As we get started, I want to acknowledge that weight is not a behavior. It is also important to be clear that there are several measures of health independent of weight. Weight is also not a reflection of any moral value of a person. Body diversity is beautiful, and body autonomy is at the forefront of my world view. And just because a diet didn't work for you doesn't mean the problem was you.

I initially decided to become a dietitian to help myself. Oh how naive to think that if only I could learn the secrets to nutrition, I would find that missing piece to solve my problems, including but not limited to my weight. (To be clear, there are no secrets.) And I learned a lot. More balanced and decidedly less restrictive, I developed a healthier—but not perfect—relationship with food. I learned the science of metabolism and calories and the magic of lean protein. I began to appreciate and consider how the social determinants of health and the systemic, institutionalized exclusion of marginalized people from equitable health care affected weight for most people. I fell in love with strength training. And, better yet, I learned how to counsel other people to eat well and, in a way, counsel myself at the same time toward a more realistic and sustainable approach to weight management.

Then, I learned about GLP-1 medications from Dr. Spencer Nadolsky. I read clinical studies. I found people online who were taking these medications. And I eventually joined Dr. Nadolsky's telehealth platform to get care for my obesity. With a BMI of 31 and a comorbidity of hypertension, and some luck with a manufacturer's coupon, I started my medication. My entire world changed, and let's be honest: It is a lot easier to work on your relationship with food, your body, and unpack the ways you were affected by diet culture when you just aren't hungry all the time.

ABOUT THIS BOOK

There are two things this book is not: an academic paper or a diet book. Both of those work in absolutes and, well, real-life nutrition for real-life people in the real world is full of nuance. What this book will cover includes:

1. Defining Obesity as a Disease
2. Everything You Need to Know About GLP-1s
3. Building a Care Team and Navigating Insurance
4. Getting Started on a GLP-1
5. Developing Your New Nutrition and Movement Philosophy
6. Eating Well and Staying Hydrated
7. Putting What You Know into Real-Life Practice
8. Sample Nutrition Plan
9. Living in the Maintenance Phase

You will also find common sense explanations of the complexity of obesity management. You'll find meal planning guidance, food lists, and sample daily menus you can use, alongside my personal perspectives, influenced by a wide breadth of context and experience in all things GLP-1s. I will do my best to be both evidence-based and realistic. My hope is that you read this and feel empowered to make your own best choices to live your healthiest life and understand the many ways (biological, environmental, and more) your situation can often be outside of your direct control. Whatever your goals, I hope we can prioritize your day-to-day quality of life along the way. So, this book is written with a few assumptions about you, reader:

- You care about your health more than the number on the scale.
- You want to feel good in your day-to-day life.
- You live in the real-ass world with real-life challenges.

PRO TIP

Establishing your *why* is an important first step before undertaking any major life change. And diving into the world of medication-assisted weight management is no minor feat. You might expect me to tell you that you need to find some sort of weight-neutral motivation, and that'll certainly help when the scale gets tricky. Please don't feel as though you have to have some secondary health-related issue to treat your obesity. Obesity itself is a metabolic disease that negatively affects quality of life for most. Having excess adipose tissue *eventually* results in poor health outcomes (more on that later). Prevention is also a perfectly acceptable motivation.

I want to make three promises to you before you read the rest of this book. I will:

1. Lead with science—no misinformation or wild claims. I discuss what I know to be true about obesity as a disease and the modern tools available to treat it.

2. Do my best to not make you feel shame or guilt about favorite foods or nutrition habits.

3. Provide actionable and useful nutrition guidance that can help you feel like your best self.

So seriously, this isn't a diet book. Diet books have rules about good and bad foods. We don't do that here. Instead, we will explore the strategies and knowledge you need to eat well *enough* to achieve your goals (whatever they may be) and live a long, healthy life, in the context of what matters to you. We eat for fun and comfort and culture *and* nutrition. We eat to live and *also* live to eat. I will focus on nutrition as a method to improve your quality of life, not just your size. *We must learn to overcome the chokehold of the number on the scale.* That's not to say we are anti–weight loss or anti-diet or anti-whatever is politically incorrect about nutrition at this time in space. Clearly, we are going to talk about weight loss and obesity and the risks and benefits of intentional weight loss. But it's not *all* about weight. Let me be very clear: It's okay to want to lose weight *to be less fat*; to soak in the positive attention and thin privilege and societal currency that comes with socially desirable aesthetics; and to look at yourself in the mirror and be like, "Yeah, I did that." There is no shame here.

HOW I CAN HELP

As a registered dietitian specializing in weight management using GLP-1 medications (and taking one myself), I'd like to share with you the knowledge and practical tips you'll need to live your healthiest life along your weight loss journey! If you're wondering how this book will help you, let's start with some of the common issues I've seen over the years . . .

Eating more whole food sources of protein and fewer from supplements. Whole protein foods from a variety of sources ensure you are consuming all of the essential amino acids in varying amounts. Different protein foods also provide a variety of nutrients, such as B vitamins, iron, magnesium, and zinc (depending on the source) that serve important roles in the body above and beyond the "protein" component.

Adding more carbs to meals for energy and side effect management. When you are living in a body with insulin resistance, lower-carbohydrate diets can be effective for weight loss and improved blood sugar control. But one reason GLP-1s are so effective for weight loss and health is that they actually improve your body's ability to use carbohydrates for energy and prevent you from storing excess calories as fat so easily. And, as a dietitian working with people taking GLP-1s, the primary reason for a visit is a side effect complaint. Fatigue, nausea, and constipation are the top three and almost always resolved by increasing carbohydrate intake. I recommend ½- to 1-cup (weight varies) portions of complex carbohydrates with every meal, three meals per day. So, adding foods such as potatoes, beans, whole grain bread products, rice, pasta, and oatmeal can improve how you feel and support healthy weight loss. Plus, adding carbohydrates to meals makes them more filling and satisfying and helps you build habits around sustainable balanced meals that serve you for a lifetime.

Lowering dietary fats by limiting portion sizes of foods such as avocado, cheese, fatty proteins, nuts, oils, peanut butter, and salad dressings. Dietary fats, even the healthy ones, tend to be the number-one cause of gastrointestinal-related side effects while on a GLP-1 medication. Dietary fats can also slow gastric emptying and contribute to feeling too full for too long. Aside from contributing to nausea, high-fat foods are also high-calorie foods. If weight loss has been slow or frustrating, an audit of your daily dietary fat intake can be revealing. I'd much rather you double your servings of carbohydrates than fats. I also recommend using the low-fat or fat-free versions of foods you use often such as dairy products and salad dressings.

Not skipping meals or waiting until you're "hungry" to eat—your new hungry may take a while to recognize. It is important to eat enough. The biggest concern when using GLP-1 medications is rapid weight loss at the expense of muscle and bone. Your daily energy and overall health depend on fueling your body. I recommend following regularly scheduled meal plans, ideally breakfast, lunch, and dinner every day, regardless of hunger. Eating daily around the same predictable time helps your body learn your new hunger and fullness cues. Learning *how much* to eat is also a skill you may need to practice, and scheduled meals can help. Of course, if you're hungry sooner than planned, eat—but reflect on how to improve the previous meal so it's more satisfying.

Stop trying to lose weight as quickly as possible—slow and steady is more sustainable. Slow and steady weight loss is maintained more easily for the long term. I recommend targeting ½ to 1 percent of starting body weight of loss per week. So, if you started your weight loss on a GLP-1 at 220 pounds (99.8 kg), an average weight loss goal of 1.1 to 2.2 pounds (0.5 to 1 kg) per week is PLENTY.

Undereating can negatively affect sleep, energy, digestion, and the ability to maintain a healthy immune system. It takes time to *learn and practice* new skills related to health, like meal planning, grocery shopping, cooking, exercising, overcoming barriers, and navigating challenges. Instead of focusing on the scale to judge progress, practice eating as much as necessary to feel your best, improving your overall diet quality, and shifting your body composition for the better.

I'm glad you are here. You don't have to do this alone. Before we dig in any deeper, a reminder: *This book is not a substitute for medical advice from your prescribers or personal health care providers*. Chapter 3 discusses how to find a care team with your best interests in mind.

The diet industry has broken our trust, and I hope you are skeptical of everything you read. Misinformation is ubiquitous, especially around GLP-1s. So, I hope in this book I am able to offer you some food for thought around obesity and our culture, level set with evidence-based, common sense nutrition guidance, and provide useful tools to help you feel your best and find your healthiest self.

INTRODUCTION: GLP-1s CHANGED MY LIFE

I was always the big girl who wanted seconds at every meal. I cannot remember a time when I was not chronically overeating as a child—I even snuck food into my room at night. And my first commercial diet program was at age sixteen. I remember then seeing 199 pounds (99.3 kg) on the scale my freshman year of high school, wanting desperately in those early 2000s to be able to wear low-rise jeans like my skinny friends and begging my mother for help. I was a high-achieving perfectionist who strived to do everything right, so naturally I wanted to eat right too! My mom, a physical education coach, also struggled with her weight. So, we looked up the next Saturday weight-loss meeting in town, and we did it together.

I learned some valuable nutrition skills in those meetings. At the time, I was knee deep into diet culture, as was our entire society back then, with a strong focus on restriction. We wrote down everything we ate in our journals to show our leader at the end of the week. The calorie restriction and increasing amounts of fruits and veggies worked. I saw 170 pounds (77.1 kg) going into sophomore year, got myself a boyfriend, and did so well that season on the basketball team that I made the newspaper! But I was still bigger than my friends. I had no model for tall muscular women being desirable—except Serena Williams, and we all remember how the media was talking about her body. I wanted to be smaller, but keeping the weight off became increasingly more difficult the harder I tried. Eventually you stop being so attentive to your nutrition. My senior-year boyfriend's family kept a fridge in their garage full of regular sodas and cookie dough. My skinny boyfriend ate like a teenage boy and, well, so did I. You see, my mother never kept those sorts of foods in our home. I also had a car and some money of my own and no one to tell me I couldn't go to McDonald's before basketball practice. And don't get me started on that $1 USD bag of chocolate chip cookies for sale every day in the cafeteria. *The food called to me no matter how much I knew I didn't need it.* By graduation, I had gained back all the weight I had lost and then some, weighing in at 220 pounds (99.8 kg) and needing an XL-size cap and gown.

I spent my college years continuing to gain weight at a rapid pace despite the occasional crash diet attempts. Cabbage soup, anyone? I had introduced alcohol on a regular basis, had access to 24/7 food hall buffets thanks to my meal plan, and lived alone where no one could see me bring in yet another fast-food meal at 3 a.m. The food-rich environment proved too difficult for me to resist. I struggled—hard—not just with my weight, but with much more than is relevant to this topic. I graduated, just barely, this time at 300 pounds

(136 kg) in an XXL-size cap and gown. I remember the difficulty I had shopping for a dress for graduation. But the best part of that day—perhaps the strongest memory—was the fried grouper sandwich I had with my family afterward.

There was a time in my early twenties when I think I was just existing, mostly just eating and existing. I was working a job that didn't pay much, letting my parents mostly support me, dating awful people, and eventually—briefly—getting fed up enough with myself to try to lose weight, again. About that time, a medical event rocked my world, and you could say I found some fear-based motivation to manage my health. I made some incremental changes that stuck. A brief moment in Overeaters Anonymous (OA) had me searching for a higher power (she was never found), then, my Forks Over Knives vegan era paired with marathon training, followed closely by my CrossFit paleo phase. Somehow, over a few years, I had actually lost 100 pounds (45.3 kg)! Nutrition had become my entire personality, and I decided to pursue a second degree to become a registered dietitian at age twenty-five. I got married, bought a house, made a baby, and took a little break from school.

Yup, a pregnancy. That first one was a doozy! I was so sick I could barely function. Then, once that resolved, it felt like it was my full-time job to eat. And did I EAT. I gained 50 pounds (22.7 kg) by the time I gave birth to my daughter—which, honestly, I wasn't too worried about. I told myself, "I know how to lose weight, right?" I rejoined a diet program at six weeks postpartum, because . . . of course. Why I felt inclined to immediately manage my weight postpartum could be its own commentary on society's pressure on women's bodies—especially new moms. Like a ton of bricks, postpartum depression nearly took me out, adding another 30 or so pounds (13.6 kg) along the way. It took me more than a year to claw myself out of it.

Somehow, I think through the sheer force of my stubbornness, I was able to go back to school and finish my dietetics degree. Dietetic internships while wearing size 20 pants brought their own challenges, but I am forever grateful for my empathetic and relatable dietitian professors (who had been open about their struggles with weight). Had they been stigmatizing, judgmental, or critical, I'm not sure I could have finished the program.

I once again became a person who managed my weight and exercised as a core pillar of my personal brand. I implemented tools that helped, like counting macros and meal prepping, which seemed to be the flexible yet portion-controlled strategy that clicked for me. "The best diet is the one you can actually stick to" was my motto. It was admittedly frustrating at times and took a lot of intentionality. I shared the process on Instagram for accountability, built a community, and found purpose by helping others while also helping myself. I fought with strangers on X (formerly Twitter) when they promoted unrealistic diets. I continued to struggle with alcohol and large meals, especially on weekends, but for the most part, it was less of a roller coaster ride. I, annoyingly, made my weight management a nonnegotiable aspect of my life. *And it was, without a doubt, absolutely exhausting.*

At 200 pounds (90.7 kg), I felt pretty strong and somewhat in control of my eating, most of the time. It was fine. If a package of Oreos made their way into my home, though, I would eat the entire thing in short order! My weight would fluctuate 10 to 20 pounds (4.5 to 9 kg), but I could usually manage to make it back to what I called my "happy weight" of 200 pounds (90.7 kg). For years, I worked as a clinical dietitian in a hospital—including a bariatric surgery program—while hovering around 210 pounds (95.3 kg). I always felt like the biggest dietitian in any room of dietitians. People thought they were being nice when they told me "I carried my weight well." But I felt as though I had to really prove myself and my skills as a dietitian to be seen as competent in my job—because, unfortunately, fellow members of the health care team equated my size to my abilities and knowledge. I became more critical of and began to advocate for my patients against weight bias in the hospital.

I somehow managed to make it through a pre-midlife crisis era with lots of alcohol, a divorce, a new husband, and, eventually, a second pregnancy mostly unscathed. I won't lie, though, my weight-focused self was quite grateful for my son's full head of hair and the relentless acid reflux that helped control my tendency for overeating those nine months. How wild is that to be happy to have reflux? I lost the "baby weight" with yet another short bout of dieting. I was eating big, balanced, high-fiber meals with lots of lean protein—definitely an improvement from before! I was too busy to spend too much time on it, so I didn't beat myself up so much when I inevitably fell off track. Plus, now as a dietitian, I felt obligated to keep my weight in check. I made it back to my "happy weight" and yet was "obese." I didn't love that weight, but I didn't hate it either. I would use macro tracking intermittently to rein in some habits and kept reminding myself that being too restrictive backfires. I bought a Peloton for my birthday two months before COVID lockdown. I managed to maintain my weight, still its own challenge that takes attention, but not as much attention as trying to lose weight. I trained for a half marathon while not trying to diet, and it felt great. I told myself I was just larger-framed, athletic, that maybe the BMI didn't apply to me because I had muscles, and, for a while there, had almost resigned myself to the idea that I would always be "plus size." But the weight was an ever-present distraction to my life. As I was aging, I was getting hypertensive. Heart disease runs in my family. My father's recent open-heart surgery was difficult to witness. The pandemic had me terrified that my larger body put me at risk. And yet, additional efforts to drop below

200 pounds (90.7 kg)—above and beyond the attention it took to maintain it—were temporary and unsustainable.

You see, the thing is, I have the chronic disease of obesity. No amount of knowledge or good intentions can treat my biology. I have an insatiable appetite. Fill me up with all the lean proteins, vegetables, and fiber you can and I'm still hungry. My chronic, relentless, and progressive disease clouds my best intentions to diet and exercise. Food calls to me. I could never have "just one" of anything. I would eat in secret. I would eat past the point of physical comfort. I could eat when I was happy or sad, stressed or relaxed. I ate when I was bored. I ate when I was busy. I could eat mindlessly and also intentionally depending on the amount of mental effort I was willing to expend to fight my biology. I had a voice in my head that never stopped reminding me I could go get some food if I wanted to. Sometimes, I would fight myself about it, shame myself, and beat myself up. Sometimes, it would win. Sometimes, I'd just brush my teeth and go to bed early to try to stop thinking about food.

I had the motivation. I had all the education and resources—the gym memberships and personal trainers and the privilege to access and afford all foods. I had the time. I had social support. I would say, "Summer, you are a smart, funny, and amazing person, why the hell can't you just stop eating?" Well, you see, eventually you have to eat something. It's not like alcohol where you can attempt to just avoid it altogether (which, of course, is its own challenge). Call it internalized fatphobia or implicit bias or societal conditioning that to be healthy meant you had to be thin. Whatever it is, I had that too and continue to work through it. I would—repeatedly—attempt to "eat the right things" by whatever diet I thought at the time might be the solution, and yet, I couldn't always stop myself from overeating even those "right things." You can only fight hunger for so long. We white-knuckle against it, try to strategize around it, and try to distract ourselves from it. We even face the shame that comes with wanting to diet at all. We try the opposite approach and give ourselves permission to stop dieting and stop restricting, get in touch with our intuition about food, and escape the diet culture as best we can—only to feel worse about ourselves as our weight creeps up. And yet, hunger—moreover, that chronic disease process of obesity—would always win. Maybe not every day, but enough.

Enter Dr. Spencer Nadolsky, tweeting about GLP-1s. Spencer and I go way back. When I first became a dietitian, I appreciated his approach to nutrition on X (formerly Twitter). He was funny yet empathetic and always spot-on. He was especially critical of nutrition extremes and the "all-or-nothing" approach to food. He constantly reinforced the power of strength training. I trusted him. So, eight years later when Spencer started talking about these antiobesity medicines, I was all ears. He would share some stories from his patients' experiences, and I would find myself saying "OMG THATS ME!" He would say, "Obesity is a chronic progressive recurrent disease; obesity is not due to a lack of willpower" and that "GLP-1s help people stick to the lifestyle skills and tools they already have."

I started GLP-1 medications and sharing my experiences online, as I do with everything in my life—but I actually almost didn't. I thought, *"If all these people who have followed me all these years see I finally lost weight, and ask, what am I going to do, lie?"* Of course, there was the backlash associated with the stigma of taking medication and the false belief that all I needed to do was diet and exercise "harder"—as if that were even possible. My friends thought I was making it all up! And then they too started taking GLP-1s. Our experiences have been nearly universal. Suddenly, that food noise that consumed my entire brain at all hours of the day was gone.

I tweeted Spencer—"Okay, this is wild, my entire brain is different." Suddenly, I could eat foods I love and know are nutritious—I am a dietitian after all—and for the first time in my life, I could stop when full. After the first week, I thought, damn, even if I don't lose a single pound, the incredible benefit to my mental health and relationship with food are worth it! Let me tell you that I didn't realize how much mental space was consumed by thoughts about food until it was gone. I'm happier. I'm less anxious. I'm more patient. I'm more productive. Now, I am the type of person who can stop after one cookie. I hardly drink alcohol anymore. I've never felt so safe around food. Is this what normal people feel like with food? I never thought it was possible. I no longer track, measure, or weigh anything I eat (although to be fair, when you do some variation of that for ten-plus years, it's like you have a tracker in your brain). Now, my guesstimates are good enough! What if I had access to these medicines in my twenties?

A few months later, I tweeted Spencer again—"Hey man, y'all hiring dietitians?" And, well, here we are. I manage an incredible team of highly skilled, compassionate, empathetic dietitians delivering life-changing 1:1 nutrition counseling and developing groundbreaking nutrition content alongside obesity-informed clinicians. I'm filming podcasts, sharing my story, counseling patients, writing blogs, working from home, and absolutely loving my life. And yes, I've lost weight—I'm down to about 160 pounds (72.6 kg)—but, funny enough, I don't really care. For the first time in my life, my weight is finally just a number. I'm building muscle and getting stronger. The weight noise and the diet noise I had long held on to in my brain, along with its best friend food noise, quieted when I started my medication in 2022.

Since starting my GLP-1 medicines, I jumped feet first into this space. I have worked with thousands of people just like you and me who struggle with their weight. Many found themselves considering and eventually using these medicines with great success. I've also been posting about my experience and my work on social media and listening to others. I sought additional certifications and am proud to be a Certified Specialist in Obesity in Weight Management (CSOWM). I hope you can see how I am uniquely qualified to support you along your journey—very few dietitians have worked with people on these medicines for as long as I have!

Beyond that, I hope you know I care—not only about your physical health, weight loss goals, and medication journey, but also about who you are as a person in this world. In this book, we will explore the science of obesity, the ways our environments and behaviors play a role in the condition, and the incredible ways these medicines work. We will explore practical, realistic, and science-backed mindset, nutrition, and fitness strategies. I hope you read this book and walk away empowered—as I am—to live a life where food is not some scary thing that needs to be restricted, but where nutrition fuels you to live your best life.

CHAPTER 01

DEFINING OBESITY AS A DISEASE

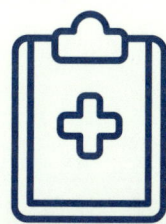

O besity is not a slur or a dirty word; it is a multifaceted health condition that has become a global epidemic, affecting millions worldwide. Obesity is a chronic, relapsing, and progressive disease, and its prevalence is worsening. Understanding its causes and effects can help us take a comprehensive approach to managing obesity without falling prey to misinformation or stigma. So, let's set the stage, build context, and ensure we are on the same page when defining obesity as a disease.

Far from being a simple matter of personal choice, managing obesity requires coordinated action on multiple fronts to create environments and tools that make a "healthy lifestyle" achievable. The mantra "eat less, move more" suggests that obesity is solely a result of individual failure, neglecting the biological, societal, and environmental factors that lead to overeating and physical inactivity, further marginalizing those struggling with obesity and perpetuating stigma.

MEDICAL CAUSES OF OBESITY

Drug-induced: Anticonvulsants, antidepressants, antipsychotics, beta blockers, contraceptives, glitazones, glucocorticoids, insulin, sulfonylureas

Endocrine: Growth hormone deficiency, hypothyroidism, pseudohypoparathyroidism

Genetic disorders: Leptin receptor (LEPR) deficiency, melanocortin 4 receptor (MC4R) deficiency, proopiomelanocortin (POMC) deficiency

Neurologic: Brain injury, brain tumor, cranial irradiation, hypothalamic obesity

Psychological: Binge eating disorder, depression

Syndromes: Alström, Bardet-Biedl (BBS), Cohen, Cushing's, Fröhlich, Prader-Willi (PWS)

OBESITY IS CHRONIC, RELAPSING, AND PROGRESSIVE

Obesity is chronic. It persists over time and requires ongoing management. Many of us have struggled with weight management for decades, since childhood perhaps. Despite various attempts at popular diets or exercise programs, most people living with obesity find it challenging to maintain a healthy weight. The biological, emotional, and environmental factors contributing to obesity are often deeply rooted and persistent, making the journey to a healthier weight a long-term challenge, to say the least.

Obesity is relapsing. Most people regain weight after losing it initially. The cycle of weight loss and regain can be discouraging. Maintenance is, arguably, more challenging than the initial weight loss itself. Weight loss triggers biological responses that fight back, including increased appetite. The cyclical nature of weight gain and loss is sensitive to environmental or emotional triggers and social and lifestyle factors that can lead to recurrent weight gain—even more reason for comprehensive support beyond dieting.

Obesity is progressive—untreated obesity (and living with excess adiposity) usually worsens health conditions as we age. I cannot emphasize enough the importance of early intervention. Youth is an amazing thing, and perhaps that is why so many people delay managing obesity until later in life. The longer we live in a body carrying excess weight, the greater the risks for a decline in health and overall quality of life.

THE CULTURE OF OBESITY BIAS

Obesity bias grows from negative stereotypes and discriminatory beliefs directed at individuals living with obesity, leading to decreased quality of life, social exclusion, and mental health challenges—exacerbating the very conditions it seeks to criticize. Media representation plays a significant role in perpetuating these biases; the portrayal of obesity is often unflattering and linked to undesirable traits such as laziness or lack of discipline, whereas thinness is equated with success, beauty, and happiness. This societal conditioning not only shapes people's perspectives but also influences health care providers' attitudes toward patients. To address obesity bias, we need to build a culture of empathy, acceptance, and understanding. By engaging in discussions and challenging our beliefs about body image and health, we create a more supportive environment where individuals are valued, irrespective of their size.

CURRENT PREVALENCE OF OBESITY

The prevalence, or how common something is within a population, of obesity among US adults stands alarmingly high and is worsening. According to the Centers for Disease Control and Prevention (CDC), during the period 2017 to 2018, about 43 percent of all US adults aged twenty and over were classified as obese (BMI > 30); this translates to roughly 100 million people and marked a significant increase from previous decades, with only 30 percent of adults classified as obese in the period 1999 to 2000.

Obesity prevalence tends to increase with age, peaking in middle-aged adults, with those aged forty to fifty-nine years having the highest prevalence. Significant disparities also exist across racial and ethnic groups; Black adults exhibit the highest obesity prevalence at about 50 percent, followed by Hispanic adults at 45 percent, white adults at 42 percent, and Asian adults at 17 percent. Black women have notably higher obesity rates (56.9 percent) compared to Black men (37.6 percent).

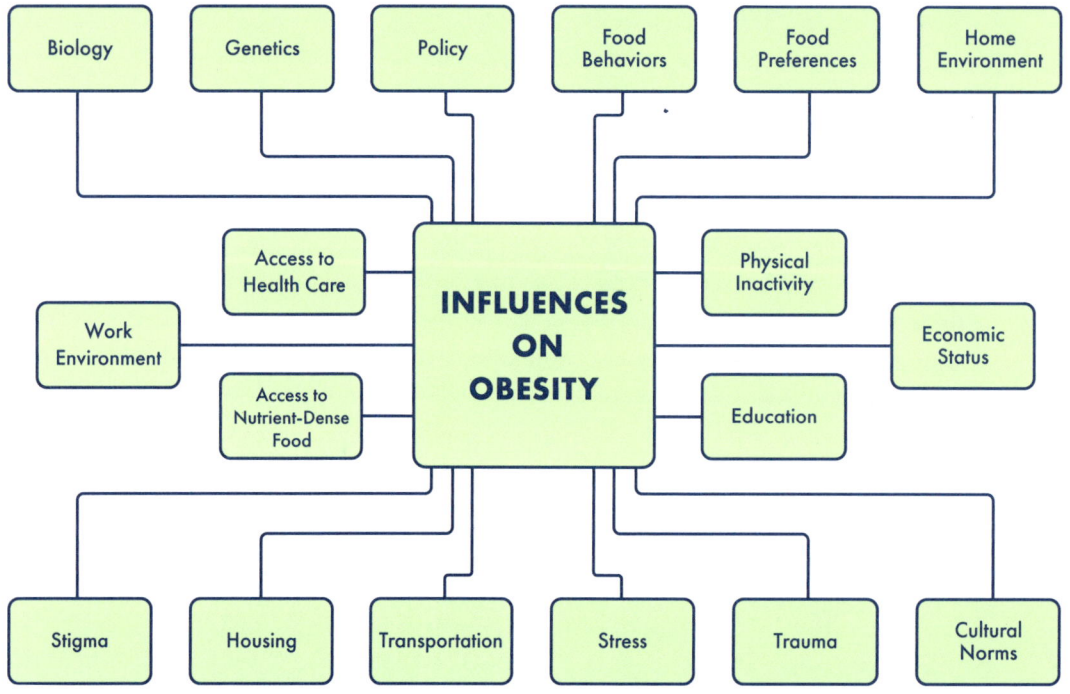

Biology • Genetics • Policy • Food Behaviors • Food Preferences • Home Environment

Access to Health Care • Work Environment • Access to Nutrient-Dense Food

INFLUENCES ON OBESITY

Physical Inactivity • Economic Status • Education

Stigma • Housing • Transportation • Stress • Trauma • Cultural Norms

MULTIFACTORIAL CAUSES OF OBESITY

It is essential to understand and recognize the complexity of obesity's causes, which include biological, environmental, political, and social influences. Far too often we blame ourselves for struggling with our weight. Although individual choices play a role in health outcomes, these choices are heavily influenced by the conditions in which we are born, grow, live, work, and age. Access to nutritious food, health care, safe environments for physical activity, and education all shape our health behaviors. When healthy options are scarce or unattainable, it's unrealistic to expect individuals to thrive. It's crucial to recognize that socioeconomic status, employment opportunities, housing, and transportation can affect someone's ability to maintain a healthy weight. *Our environment and biology interact in complex ways to shape our behavior.* High-stress environments, for instance, can lead to hormonal changes that increase appetite and fat storage. Genetics and early-life nutrition can predispose individuals to weight gain. By understanding that behaviors are not simply a matter of willpower but a response to our biological makeup and environmental conditions, we can foster more empathy for ourselves and others while looking for solutions to the actual problems.

BIOLOGICAL INFLUENCES ON OBESITY

Biological factors—genetics, metabolic processes, and physiology—play a critical role in the development of obesity. Although it's difficult to pinpoint just one particular gene for all, it's likely an interplay of the expression of thousands of different genes that affect the way our body works, including hunger, satiety, and fat storage. Our metabolic rate, the rate at which the body burns calories, varies greatly from person to person. Basal metabolic rate (BMR), which accounts for the largest portion of daily caloric expenditure, is influenced by factors such as age, sex, and muscle mass. Hormones such as leptin, insulin, and ghrelin play crucial roles in regulating body weight. Leptin, produced by fat cells, helps regulate energy balance by inhibiting hunger. However, in obese individuals, leptin resistance can occur, meaning that despite high levels of leptin in the body, the brain does not respond adequately, leading to increased hunger and food intake. Insulin resistance, often associated with obesity, can also disrupt normal metabolic processes and contribute to weight gain. Significant weight loss leads to reductions in leptin and increases in ghrelin, which increases appetite, driving weight regain.

SOCIAL AND ENVIRONMENTAL INFLUENCES ON OBESITY

The modern lifestyle often promotes unhealthy dietary habits and sedentary behavior. The food environment encourages the intake of highly palatable high-calorie foods, often high in sugars and unhealthy fats, which contributes to excessive caloric intake and weight gain. Physical inactivity due to sedentary occupations, reliance on personal vehicles for transportation, increased screen time, and limited access to recreational facilities reduces caloric expenditure, which can result in weight gain over time. Financial constraints may lead to the consumption of cheaper, energy-dense foods with limited nutritional value, which also promotes weight gain. Psychological aspects such as trauma, stress, mental health, and emotional well-being can also influence eating behaviors and physical activity levels.

Emotional eating, often triggered by stress or psychological distress, can lead to overconsuming high-calorie foods and the subsequent weight gain.

CULTURAL AND COMMUNITY INFLUENCES ON OBESITY

Cultural norms and community environments also shape dietary behaviors and attitudes toward food and physical activity. In some cultures, higher body weight may be associated with prosperity and health whereas in others, higher body weights are stigmatized and discriminated against, influencing personal and community attitudes toward weight. I would be remiss not to acknowledge the intersections of weight issues with economic and health care disparities seen in genders and races. Historically and systematically, excluded and marginalized groups have a steeper hill to climb. Social networks also affect lifestyle choices, as individuals tend to mirror the behaviors of peers and family members.

POLITICAL INFLUENCES ON OBESITY

Policies, legislation, and political decisions at the local, national, and international levels can both mitigate and exacerbate obesity rates. If we are going to promote effective and equitable strategies to combat obesity, politics are, for better or worse, part of the picture. Decisions regarding agricultural subsidies can influence the availability and affordability of certain foods, often disproportionately allocated to crops like corn, soy, and wheat, which are primary ingredients in processed foods, resulting in calorie-dense foods in stores that are more affordable and accessible compared to fresh fruits, meats, and vegetables.

Policies that mandate clear and transparent food labeling can empower consumers to make healthier choices but also confuse and shift our focus away from what really matters (looking at you, non-GMO labels on things that could never be GMO).

Governments can also regulate the marketing of foods. Taxation on unhealthy foods and beverages (in the same way we tax alcohol and tobacco, for example) has been implemented in several regions with mixed results. Revenue from these taxes can be reinvested into public health initiatives, including nutrition education and community health programs. However, it is essential to design these taxes so they do not disproportionately burden low-income individuals who may already face economic challenges and to discuss them in a way that doesn't demonize certain foods.

The extent to which governments prioritize obesity as a public health issue often vacillates between nonexistent and overbearing. Policies and interventions to reduce obesity require sustained commitment and funding, as the issues surrounding obesity are not easily solved in a single election cycle. A well-informed and accurate recognition of obesity's impact on health care costs and population health could drive comprehensive and long-term strategies. Advocacy can be instrumental in highlighting inequities and driving policy changes that promote health equity. Grassroots movements and nongovernmental organizations can mobilize public support and put pressure on policymakers to implement evidence-based strategies for obesity prevention and management.

Political decisions regarding urban planning and the infrastructure of our built environments affect community physical activity levels. Equitable distribution of resources and facilities is essential to ensure all communities have opportunities for healthy living. Investments in public transportation, pedestrian-friendly streets, parks, and recreation facilities encourage active living. Conversely, neglecting urban planning in marginalized communities can influence physical inactivity and create higher obesity rates. Schools are also crucial settings for shaping children's dietary behaviors and physical activity patterns, and it is political decisions that drive the management of school meal programs, physical education requirements, and the availability of nutritious food in school cafeterias.

Access to health care services, including preventive care and treatment for obesity, is also influenced by political decisions about health care policy and funding. Universal health care coverage and policies that integrate obesity prevention and management into primary care—and appropriately reimburse providers for doing so—can ensure equitable access to necessary services. Improving access and coverage for nutrition counseling from registered dietitians is shown to improve outcomes. Addressing systemic barriers within the health care system, such as stigma and bias against individuals with obesity, requires not just cultural or social movements but also political shifts in understanding.

HEALTH CARE INDUSTRY INFLUENCES ON OBESITY

The health care system, which should be a useful resource for individuals seeking to improve their health, is not immune to biases and inequities concerning weight. Research consistently shows that individuals with higher body weights face significant disparities in accessing quality health care services. Access to evidence-based obesity care is often limited by socioeconomic status, race, and geography. Health care providers need better education on obesity and training to deliver compassionate, individualized care. Implicit biases and overt fatphobia in health care not only undermine the therapeutic relationship but also harm patients; studies reveal that providers who hold antifat biases may unintentionally deliver lower quality care or offer unhelpful weight-related advice. Patients with obesity often experience "diagnostic overshadowing," where clinicians attribute all health issues to weight rather than addressing the individual holistically. This approach can result in misdiagnoses and unaddressed health problems. Asking your provider to consider how they would treat a person who is not living with obesity for the same complaints may reveal surprising answers.

Despite a growing body of research supporting various evidence-based interventions for obesity, barriers to access remain prevalent. As with many aspects of public health, privilege plays a significant role in accessing health care resources and treatment for obesity. Policies that seek to address these barriers genuinely must focus on expanding insurance coverage for obesity treatments. By advocating for policies that prioritize diversity in body types and treat obesity as a complex health issue rather than a moral failing, we can collectively move toward a more equitable health care landscape.

FOOD INDUSTRY INFLUENCES ON OBESITY

The food industry plays a significant role in shaping dietary habits and, by extension, obesity rates. The industry's practices, dominated by profit motives, often prioritize convenience and palatability over nutritional value. The manipulation of food ingredients to prolong shelf life and enhance flavors often results in less nutritious options dominating the market, contributing to higher caloric intake and obesity. The omnipresence of fast food and convenience items makes it challenging for individuals to maintain a balanced diet, particularly in environments termed "food deserts," where access to fresh foods is limited. Highly processed foods, often high in sugars, fats, and salts to enhance taste and increase sales, are produced at large scale, making them cheaper and more readily available than fresher, more nutritious options. These additives can make foods more enjoyable, encouraging overconsumption.

The food industry spends billions on advertising to promote its products, which exerts a significant influence on dietary behaviors, often encouraging the consumption of less nutritious or satiating foods. Advertisements often highlight highly processed foods and sugary beverages, making them appear more desirable. Techniques such as celebrity endorsements, appealing visuals, and emotional messaging create positive associations with these products. With the rise of digital media, food advertising has expanded to online platforms. Social media influencers, targeted ads, and sponsored content further normalize the consumption of unhealthy foods. Digital marketing can be particularly insidious, as it exploits algorithms to customize ads based on individual preferences and behaviors.

Economic barriers often dictate the affordability and accessibility of healthier food options, such as fresh fruits, vegetables, and lean proteins, which also tend to be more expensive than processed and fast foods. For individuals and families with limited financial resources, economic constraints can create a reliance on cheaper, calorie-dense, nutrient-poor foods, exacerbating higher obesity rates among low-income populations. Food insecurity, the lack of stable access to sufficient food, is paradoxically linked to obesity.

FOOD PREFERENCE INFLUENCES ON OBESITY

Food preferences, shaped by cultural, social, industrial, and individual factors, may be one of the strongest influences on dietary behaviors. *Simply put, if you don't like it, you probably won't eat it.* Early exposure to sugary, fatty, and salty foods can create lasting preferences that are hard to change. Biologically, humans are predisposed to prefer sweet, salty, and fatty tastes. Foods that are satiating and health-promoting with high levels of fiber and protein are often not as appealing unless prepared well. The food industry's formulation of highly palatable processed foods amplifies these natural preferences, making healthier choices less appealing by comparison. Efforts to modify taste preferences through gradual exposure to healthier foods and developing cooking skills can help shift dietary habits over time.

RISKS OF OBESITY

Living with obesity poses significant risks to physical health, mental well-being, and overall quality of life, especially as we age. There is some argument as to whether it is the lack of health-promoting lifestyle habits, like a nutritious diet or physical activity, that increases obesity's risks or if it is the biological impact of the excess adipose tissue itself. But like all things health, it's not an either-or scenario. I'd argue that our increased risks for poor health related to our lifestyle choices and body size (in the context of all the other relevant social determinants of health) simply compound over time.

- Obesity—living with excess adiposity—directly increases the risk for cardiovascular diseases.

- Excess body fat can cause the kidneys to retain sodium, leading to increased blood pressure. Accumulation of fat, especially around the abdomen, is associated with elevated cholesterol levels, atherosclerosis, and a higher risk of coronary artery disease, heart attacks, and stroke.

- Excess weight, particularly visceral fat (the fat stored around the internal organs), impairs the body's ability to use insulin effectively, leading to insulin resistance and an increased risk of developing type 2 diabetes.

- Obesity can contribute to obstructive sleep apnea, where airway blockage results in interrupted breathing during sleep and exacerbates asthma symptoms. High body weight places stress on joints, particularly the knees, hips, and lower back, which can lead to wear and tear and the development of osteoarthritis.

- Obesity can hinder physical activity, leading to decreased muscle mass and further physical limitations.

- Obesity is linked to an increased risk of several types of cancer, including breast, colon, endometrial, esophageal, and kidney.

- A higher prevalence of gallstones is noted in people with obesity, often due to increased cholesterol in bile.

- And lastly, for the purpose of painting this unfortunate picture, but certainly not least, excess body weight can increase abdominal pressure, leading to heartburn and acid reflux.

- Aside from the physical health concerns that arise the longer we live with a body carrying excess adipose tissue, the social and psychological effects of the disease are just as concerning.

- Mobility issues decrease physical stamina, and pain can limit participation in daily and recreational activities, leading to a reduced overall quality of life.

- The burden of obesity can lead to mental health decline, experiences of societal stigma, low self-esteem, body dissatisfaction, and social isolation.

- Obesity can sometimes coexist with or lead to eating disorders.

- Overweight and obese individuals often face bias and discrimination in various settings such as workplaces, schools, and even health care environments, which can exacerbate physical and mental health risks and lower quality of life.

- Individuals with obesity typically incur higher medical expenses due to their need for frequent medical care, medications, and interventions for obesity-related conditions later in life. These conditions are shown to result in more frequent absenteeism from work and decreased productivity, which affects both the individual's financial security and the broader economy.

UNDERSTANDING FOOD NOISE

If you have it, you know what it is. If you don't, you probably think I'm just talking about the noise people make when eating, like chewing. Misophonia is a rare condition that causes people to have strong emotional reactions to everyday sounds, such as chewing, that are usually not noticed by others—but that's not what we are talking about here.

Food noise, in the scientific community, is a relatively new term that doesn't really have a totally agreed-upon definition. There is some emerging research on the topic, though. For example, in the 2023 paper titled "What Is Food Noise? A Conceptual Model of Food Cue Reactivity" by Hayashi et al., the authors define "food noise" as the various environmental cues related to food that can influence eating behavior, even when individuals are not actively or biologically hungry. The authors aim to provide a framework to understand how these cues—such as advertising, packaging, social influences, and even the presence of food in our surroundings—can trigger cravings and lead to increased food consumption, explaining why people often eat even when they aren't physically hungry. They argue that the rise of obesity and unhealthy eating patterns is strongly related to changes to our modern food environments that are filled with constant messaging and easy access to food.

Food cues can trigger physiological responses even in the absence of hunger, involving brain regions associated with reward and craving. For instance, visual or olfactory cues can activate areas in the brain, like the nucleus accumbens and the amygdala, known to play key roles in the reward circuitry. This can increase motivation to seek out and consume food. Hormones such as ghrelin (the hunger hormone) and leptin (which signals satiety) are influenced by food cues and play essential roles in regulating appetite and body weight. When individuals encounter appealing food cues, ghrelin levels may rise, stimulating hunger even if the person has recently eaten. Conversely, continued exposure to food cues can disrupt the normal signaling of leptin, leading to an imbalance in hunger and satiety signals.

The article also discusses how the brain's reward system becomes activated in response to food cues. This activation is tied to the release of dopamine, a neurotransmitter associated with pleasure and reward. When individuals see or smell foods they enjoy, dopamine levels can increase, resulting in heightened cravings and an increased likelihood of consuming those foods. This biological process

PRO TIP

Managing food noise without medication can be tricky, but it is not impossible. Recognizing it's happening and naming it is the first step! Then, change your environment (leave the kitchen!), find distractions and activities you enjoy (go for a walk!), or even talk it out with a friend. Learning to tolerate the discomfort of food noise episodes without giving in can help you strengthen that resistance!

explains why certain food cues—especially those associated with high-calorie and palatable foods—can override personal goals related to dieting or healthy eating. The paper also touches upon how conditioning (both classical and operant) can contribute to cue reactivity. For instance, individuals may develop an association between specific environments (like a kitchen or a restaurant) and eating behaviors, leading to cravings when they encounter these environments, regardless of their physical hunger status. This conditioned response is often rooted in biological mechanisms that are influenced by past experiences with food.

Food noise, as it is known in the world of obesity medicine, is both unique to the individual and yet somehow extremely relatable to those of us who suffer from it. I think everyone, even without obesity, has cues that are not entirely biological that trigger them to want to eat. Everyone has cravings—it's very human to see very tasty food and want to eat it. It's also a very responsible adult activity to plan your meals and look forward to eating something appealing. What's not "normal," though, is thinking about food constantly in a way that distracts you from everything else and negatively affects your ability to manage your weight and nutrition in a healthy way.

People who do not struggle with food noise are able to eat their usual foods and simply move on. For me, though, food noise often felt like a relentless background soundtrack I couldn't turn down, influencing all of my food choices and constantly **interfering** with my daily life. It's the mental gymnastics around nutrition management that only get louder the more you try to resist. It's that voice in your head that doesn't shut up about food. And if you aren't thinking about eating, you're thinking about starting your next diet or how what you eat will affect your

FOOD CUES

External
- Senses
- Environment
- Social

Internal
- Hunger
- Thoughts
- Energy

CONSTANT INFLUENCERS

- Genes
- Body size
- Appetite
- Food preferences
- Emotional skills
- Medical conditions

TRANSIENT INFLUENCERS

- Time
- Place
- Activity
- Sleep
- Stress
- Emotional state
- Hormonal state

FOOD CUE REACTIVITY

Biological Changes
- Heart rate
- Blood pressure
- Body temperature
- Gastric activity
- Brain activity
- Salivation

Psychological Changes
- Attention and focus
- Food noise and cravings
- Anticipation of reward
- Anticipation of relief
- Awareness of physical hunger
- Thoughts of food

OUTCOMES

Short-term
- Food-seeking behaviors
- Increased food intake
- Reward and pleasure
- Distress and disappointment

Long-term
- Weight gain
- Disordered eating
- Decreased quality of life
- Incentive sensitization
- Classical conditioning
- Operant conditioning

Image adapted from "What Is Food Noise? A Conceptual Model of Food Cue Reactivity" by Hayashi et al. with modifications.

KEY TERMS

Incentive sensitization: Your brain becomes more sensitive to certain foods, making you *crave* them more. Over time, you may feel a strong desire to eat those foods, even if they don't taste as amazing as they once did.

Classical conditioning (Pavlovian learning): Your brain connects a specific cue or environment to eating, so you automatically feel like eating when the cue is present, even if you're not hungry.

Operant conditioning: You learn to eat certain foods or behave a certain way around food based on rewards (feeling of joy, energy) or consequences (upset stomach).

weight (I call those "diet noise" and "weight noise," food noise's evil twins) as a way to compensate for all the eating you've already done.

The food noise in my head and the behaviors that ensued went a little something like this . . .

- Every morning, my first thoughts revolved around food and weight

- Actively eating breakfast while thinking about dinner

- Being unable to leave the house without stopping for coffee and a treat

- Waiting until no one was watching to go back for additional helpings

- Remembering every major life event based on the food consumed (and my weight)—not the people or conversations

- White-knuckling past fast-food restaurants on my commutes or giving in and having fast food in secret, then eating dinner later with my family

- Knowing, by heart, every menu item at every common fast-food or chain restaurant

- And having very specific orders for "healthy times" versus "whatever times"

- Feeling like anything high in sugar had to be completely banned from my home, or otherwise it "called to me"

- Eating past the point of comfort in any scenario with unlimited food—buffets, cruises, football parties, Thanksgiving

- Inability to resist treats and snacks at work—even those leftover stale ones

- Heightened anxiety at restaurants, overthinking my choices, and somehow still "ordering wrong"

- Needing to know the "food situation" before going anywhere or doing anything, with extreme anxiety not knowing what foods would be available and when

- Seeing a commercial or social media post about a certain food, then obsessing about how, when, and where to get that food—sometimes for days

- Struggling to resist the candy bars in the grocery store's checkout line

- Stealing food from other people—"just a taste" of my husband's plate at a restaurant; those cold, dry chicken nuggets my kids didn't want; Mommy tax on those french fries

- Buying way too much food when grocery shopping, including a pack of raw cookie dough, which I ate in the parking lot before driving home

- Standing in the kitchen after the kids go to bed eating one of everything possible trying to satisfy a very unspecific craving—and going to bed still hungry

- Negotiating with myself for permission to indulge: working out harder or longer or skipping the next meal, which never worked out

Thankfully, GLP-1s turned off that noise—for the most part. It's amazing how much more you can do and think about when you aren't thinking just about food all the time! I'm forever grateful for getting the brain space back.

CHAPTER 02

EVERYTHING YOU NEED TO KNOW ABOUT GLP-1s

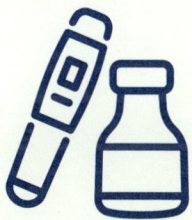

Now that we understand that obesity is a disease and very much not your fault, let's learn about our options for managing it. We will start with a brief look at the history of dieting and obesity treatments of the past—many you've probably tried! Then, we will dive headfirst into learning about the exciting and revolutionary new obesity treatments, called GLP-1 receptor agonists, that are dominating our culture and health care space.

We will explore how these new medications work to improve glucose regulation and appetite control, resulting in clinically significant weight loss and improved health. For simplicity's sake, I generally refer to these medications as "GLP-1s," even though there are many different medications in this category, as they all tend to work in many of the same ways, but we'll also look at some of their differences.

Before we get started, just to be sure we are all on the same page, these are the medicines I discuss in this book:

- The GLP-1 agonist semaglutide, with brand names Ozempic and Wegovy
- The GLP-1/GIP dual agonist tirzepatide, with brand names Mounjaro and Zepbound

DIETING AND OBESITY TREATMENT IN AMERICA BEFORE GLP-1s

The pursuit of weight loss in the United States has a long and complex history, shaped by cultural, social, and scientific influences, from early dietary practices to the introduction of pharmaceutical interventions. In the early nineteenth century, obesity was often viewed as a symptom of excess and self-indulgence. In the early twentieth century, the boom of print publications birthed a wide variety of weight management–related resources, just like the grifters and gurus that seem to keep popping up with new and exciting approaches to nutrition online: intermittent fasting, low-carb, and extremely low-calorie approaches were "new" then.

1960s

The 1960s saw the introduction of the Weight Watchers program (founded in 1963), which focused on community support, good and bad foods, weight monitoring, and portion control. Weight Watchers pioneered the idea of a structured, group-oriented approach to dieting, emphasizing the importance of social interaction in achieving dieting goals.

1970s

The 1970s brought about a wave of dieting fads, including the Grapefruit Diet, the Scarsdale Diet, and the Cabbage Soup Diet, which were often extreme and unsustainable. Culturally, Cher shocked audiences showing off her bare midriff on popular television, and ultra-thin super models influenced the ideal aesthetic.

1980s

By the 1980s, obesity in America had been recognized as an epidemic, leading to more significant public health initiatives aimed at combating weight gain. Throughout the 1980s, the diet industry surged with the influence of celebrity culture, print and television media, and numerous books and products.

OBESITY WORLDWIDE

Of course, obesity is not an American-only problem. The World Health Organization (WHO) reports that, in 1995, there were an estimated 200 million obese adults worldwide and another 18 million children under five classified as overweight. As of 2000, the number of obese adults had increased to more than 300 million. Contrary to conventional wisdom, the obesity epidemic is not restricted to industrialized societies; in developing countries, it is estimated that more than 115 million people suffer from obesity-related problems.

1990s

The 1990s brought us a surge in the popularity of diets like the Atkins Diet (with the book first published in the 1970s), which promoted a low carbohydrate intake. Other notable programs continued to thrive, such as Jenny Craig, which had been established in 1983, and Nutrisystem, first launched in 1972, both of which saw commercial success by offering more structured meal plans. The diet industry was booming along with the rest of the economy! The National Institutes of Health (NIH) released its first clinical guidelines for the treatment of obesity in 1998, emphasizing lifestyle changes such as diet and exercise.

2000s

Luckily, the early 2000s saw the start of the slow shift toward understanding obesity as a chronic disease rather than merely a failure of willpower. This change was vital in shaping public health strategies and funding for obesity research. The Obesity Action Coalition (OAC) was founded in 2005, providing a platform for addressing obesity through education and advocacy. Bariatric surgery also gained popularity in the early 2000s, with procedures like gastric bypass and laparoscopic adjustable gastric banding being performed more frequently. These surgical options became a viable solution for those with severe obesity when lifestyle changes and medications were ineffective. And finally, in June 2013, the American Medical Association (AMA) voted to recognize obesity as a disease (and not simply a cosmetic concern), influencing more robust research and insurance coverage for treatment and prevention efforts.

PHARMACEUTICAL OPTIONS PRE—GLP-1s

Over the years, the landscape of obesity medications has evolved, with several agents demonstrating varying mechanisms of action and safety profiles. While older medications like phentermine remain in use for short-term weight management, newer medications, such as semaglutide, have revolutionized the approach to long-term obesity treatment. Please remember that ongoing monitoring for safety and efficacy remains crucial for all approved obesity treatments. And, of course, all medications come with potential side effects. Here is a review of the pharmaceutical options that have been available for the treatment of obesity over the years.

Phentermine (Adipex-P, Ionamin)

- **First introduced:** 1959
- **Mechanism of action:** Phentermine is an appetite suppressant that stimulates the central nervous system, increasing heart rate and reducing appetite.
- **Issues:** Common side effects include increased blood pressure, insomnia, and anxiety. Due to its stimulant properties, phentermine is not recommended for long-term use because of the risk of dependence.
- **Current status:** Phentermine is still commonly prescribed for short-term weight loss and is typically part of a broader plan that includes lifestyle changes. Its relatively low cost makes it a popular short-term option for weight management.

Orlistat (Alli, Xenical)

- **First introduced:** 1999
- **Mechanism of action:** Orlistat is a lipase inhibitor that prevents fat absorption from the diet, decreasing calories absorbed.
- **Issues:** Common side effects include gastrointestinal problems such as oily stool and flatulence. It may also interfere with the absorption of fat-soluble vitamins (A, D, E, K), thus requiring supplementation.

- **Current status:** Orlistat is still available as a prescription (Xenical) and over the counter (Alli), though gastrointestinal side effects can deter some users.

Rimonabant (Acomplia)

- **First introduced:** 2006
- **Mechanism of action:** Rimonabant was an endocannabinoid receptor blocker, which helped reduce appetite and improve metabolic profiles.
- **Issues:** This drug faced significant issues due to psychological side effects, including increased risk of depression and anxiety.
- **Current status:** The drug was never approved or marketed in the United States and was withdrawn from further study in 2008 due to safety concerns regarding mental health risks.

Lorcaserin (Belviq)

- **First introduced:** 2012
- **Mechanism of action:** Lorcaserin is a selective serotonin receptor agonist that promotes feelings of fullness and reduces appetite.
- **Issues:** Safety concerns arose regarding potential cardiovascular risks and an association with certain types of cancer suggested by post-marketing studies.
- **Current status:** The US Food and Drug Administration (FDA) withdrew lorcaserin from the market in early 2020 due to safety concerns related to cancer.

Phentermine + Topiramate (Qsymia)

- **First introduced:** 2012
- **Mechanism of action:** This combination medication utilizes phentermine (an appetite suppressant) and topiramate (an anticonvulsant) to enhance weight loss through a combined effect on appetite and energy expenditure.
- **Issues:** Side effects include dry mouth, constipation, and insomnia, along with concerns about potential birth defects if used during pregnancy.
- **Current status:** Qsymia is currently available on the market and used for chronic weight management.

Naltrexone + Bupropion (Contrave)

- **First introduced:** 2014
- **Mechanism of action:** This combination medication uses naltrexone (an opioid antagonist) alongside bupropion (an antidepressant) to suppress hunger and control cravings.
- **Issues:** Side effects can include nausea, constipation, headache, and even increased risk of seizures, particularly in patients with a history of eating disorders.
- **Current status:** Contrave remains a viable option for obesity treatment and is approved for use in conjunction with lifestyle modifications.

You may notice that metformin isn't included in this discussion, and that's because it is not really a weight-loss medication. Metformin works, for very few people, as an aid in weight management by stabilizing blood sugars and improving insulin resistance somewhat, which, in theory, may help with cravings. For people with polycystic ovary syndrome, prediabetes, or diabetes, it can help improve A1C levels. So, if, by chance, you have cravings and hunger that are extremely reactive to volatile blood sugar swings, you may benefit. But, for most, this medication does very little for weight loss, as it is not an appetite suppressant.

PRO TIP

Pharmaceutical company websites are excellent resources to learn more about these medications. You will find educational videos, research papers, safety information, blogs, testimonials, FAQs, support chats, and 1-800 numbers. All the information is highly regulated and meticulously curated to improve the patient experience.

GLP-1 HISTORY AND DEVELOPMENT

As modern medicine evolved, scientists were trying to understand how the body controls blood sugar levels, particularly through the hormones released after eating. One key discovery made around the 1970s was the hormone glucagon-like peptide-1 (GLP-1), which helps regulate blood sugar by stimulating insulin release from the pancreas. This hormone in the body—the intrinsic GLP-1—is fleeting, as it increases in response to food and quickly metabolizes. Although its existence was known, at the time, there wasn't much that could be done to manipulate it in any significant way.

Fast-forward to the 1990s in the random world of reptiles, researchers discovered that a hormone similar to GLP-1 was present in a very unlikely animal: the Gila monster, a venomous lizard (dragon?!) found in the southwestern United States and Mexico. Among the substances in Gila monster venom was a peptide called exendin-4, which shares a remarkable similarity to human GLP-1. However, there were crucial differences that made exendin-4 even more appealing to pharmaceutical companies for potential use as a medicine:

- **Stability:** Unlike human GLP-1, which is quickly broken down in the body by the enzyme dipeptidyl peptidase-4, exendin-4 is resistant to degradation. This means it lasts much longer in the bloodstream, extending its biological effects.

- **Potency:** Exendin-4 effectively binds to the same receptors as GLP-1, making it a powerful stimulator of insulin release and inhibitor of glucagon secretion.

One key figure in this journey was Dr. John Eng, an endocrinologist at the Veterans Affairs Medical Center in New York. He recognized exedin-4's potential as a treatment for diabetes because it could mimic the effects of human GLP-1 but with a longer duration of action. In the early 2000s, pharmaceutical companies saw the potential of exendin-4 and started developing it into a medication. This led to the creation of the first GLP-1 receptor agonist, a twice-daily injectable called exenatide (brand name Byetta), which was approved for use in 2005.

The success of exenatide spurred interest in creating additional GLP-1 receptor agonists. Several new medications have since been developed with enhancements in their pharmacokinetic properties, allowing for more convenient dosing schedules. Liraglutide was approved for diabetes in 2010, with a longer half-life, allowing for once-daily dosing. It was later approved by the FDA as Saxenda for chronic weight management in people living with obesity. Introduced in 2014, dulaglutide (brand name Trulicity) was the first of the once-weekly injections, offering patients convenience and improving adherence and outcomes. Clinical trials for these early medications have demonstrated efficacy in lowering hemoglobin A1C (HbA1c; your average blood sugar over about three months, a key marker of diabetes), inducing weight loss, and providing cardiovascular benefits. The LEADER trial (Liraglutide Effect and Action in Diabetes: Evaluation of Cardiovascular Outcome Results) showed that liraglutide significantly reduced the risk of major cardiovascular events in patients with type 2 diabetes, results so exciting that pharmaceutical companies were committed to continued improvements (and profits!). In 2017, semaglutide was approved for diabetes treatment under the brand name Ozempic, and in 2021, the FDA approved the same medication for obesity under the brand name Wegovy.

GLP-1 Generic Medication Name	Administration	Brand Name FDA Approved for Diabetes*	Brand Name FDA Approved for Obesity	Percent of Total Body Weight Loss Expected
Exenatide injection	Twice daily	Byetta (2005)		2 percent
Dulaglutide Injection	Once weekly	Trulicity (2014)		3 to 5 percent
Liraglutide injection	Once daily	Victoza (2010)	Saxenda (2014)	8 percent
Semaglutide injection	Once weekly	Ozempic (2017)	Wegovy (2021)	15 percent
Semaglutide oral tablet	Once daily	Rybelsus (2019)		8 percent
Tirzepatide injection (GLP-1 + GIP)	Once weekly	Mounjaro (2022)	Zepbound (2023)	20 to 25 percent

Paired with proper nutrition and exercise.
*People who have diabetes tend to lose less weight than people without diabetes.

Patient utilization of GLP-1 medications has dramatically increased since 2017, driven in part by the cultural interest in any and all things weight management. According to reports, the number of Ozempic prescriptions has skyrocketed since the drug's approval, with estimates suggesting more than three million prescriptions were filled in the United States alone by 2023. Following its launch in June 2021, Wegovy quickly gained traction, with more than one million prescriptions reported within its first year on the market. But 2022 wasn't great for Wegovy: Manufacturing issues plagued this medication and made if nearly impossible to find in pharmacies. Tirzepatide had a boom year in 2022 when Mounjaro hit the market with an attractive manufacturer coupon and took the internet by storm. By 2023, however, Wegovy exceeded two million prescriptions in the United States. Early estimates indicated that Mounjaro and Zepbound were rapidly accruing a significant number of prescriptions, exceeding the three million patients actively using these therapies in the United States alone in 2024.

Although it may sound like "everyone is using these medications," knowing that, according to the US Centers for Disease Control, there are nearly one hundred million people living with obesity in the United States, there are many more who may benefit from this treatment who are not yet able to access it.

INTERNATIONAL CONSIDERATIONS FOR OBESITY TREATMENT

Obesity has emerged as a significant international health concern, transcending borders and affecting populations across the globe. According to the World Health Organization (WHO), worldwide obesity has nearly tripled since 1975, with alarming rates seen in both developed and developing nations. This increase is attributed to several interrelated factors, including urbanization, changes in dietary patterns, and a decline in physical activity levels. As countries industrialize and urbanize, traditional diets rich in whole foods are often replaced by processed foods high in sugars and fats, leading to poor nutritional choices.

One major driver of rising obesity rates is the globalization of food markets. Fast-food chains and processed food brands have penetrated diverse markets, making calorie-dense, nutrient-poor foods more accessible and appealing. Additionally, the rise of sedentary lifestyles, fueled by technological advancements and urban living means that physical activity levels have plummeted. With more people engaging in desk jobs and leisure activities centered on screens, the balance between calorie intake and expenditure has shifted unfavorably.

The landscape of GLP-1 medications, primarily used for managing type 2 diabetes and obesity, varies significantly across international markets outside the United States. Countries in Europe, Canada, and Australia have been at the forefront of adopting these medications, generally providing access to these therapies within the same year they become available in the United States. In Europe, for example, several GLP-1 receptor agonists, such as liraglutide and semaglutide, are available and have gained approval from regulatory bodies such as the European Medicines Agency (EMA) and are often included in national health care plans, making them more accessible to patients.

Cost considerations for GLP-1 medications differ widely depending on the country. In Canada, for instance, these drugs are generally covered under provincial health plans, but patients may face out-of-pocket expenses if they don't meet certain clinical criteria, such as specific BMI thresholds for obesity treatment. In contrast, countries such as Germany and France provide broader access through public health insurance, though there can still be variations in reimbursement based on regional health policies. On the other hand, patients in countries with less comprehensive health care systems may see higher out-of-pocket costs, making these medications less accessible.

Differing requirements for obtaining GLP-1 medications also reflect each country's health care philosophy and economic conditions. In some countries, strict guidelines ensure that only patients with severe obesity or poorly controlled diabetes are prescribed these medications, whereas others may allow broader access based on patient preference or physician recommendation. For example, in the United Kingdom, the National Institute for Health and Care Excellence (NICE) has specific guidelines that dictate eligibility for obesity treatment, influencing how easily patients can obtain these drugs. This disparity often stems from local health care budgets and the cost-effectiveness evaluations that each health authority conducts, balancing the benefits of these medications against their financial implications.

Beyond their proven benefits for diabetes management, GLP-1 receptor agonists are being explored for several other therapeutic applications:

- **Cardiovascular health:** Numerous studies (especially for semaglutide) indicate that GLP-1 receptor agonists not only help with glycemic control but also offer cardiovascular protection, reducing the risks of heart attacks and strokes.

- **Cognitive disorders:** There is emerging interest in exploring the potential neuroprotective effects of GLP-1 receptor agonists for conditions such as Alzheimer's disease, though this research is in its early stages, thought in part to be beneficial due to anti-inflammatory benefits for the brain.

- **Nonalcoholic steatohepatitis and liver disease:** Ongoing research looks at the potential benefits of GLP-1 receptor agonists in treating these conditions due to their effects on weight, insulin sensitivity, and lipid metabolism.

- **Obesity treatment:** GLP-1 receptor agonists promote satiety and reduce food intake, making them effective for weight management.

- **Polycystic ovarian syndrome and menopause:** Many women with polycystic ovarian syndrome struggle with weight gain and obesity, which can exacerbate the syndrome's symptoms. By reducing insulin resistance, GLP-1 medications can help normalize a variety of hormone levels, which may improve menstrual regularity and reduce androgen levels, alleviating symptoms like hirsutism (excessive hair growth) and acne. Menopause, similarly, increases insulin resistance and increases the risk of cardiovascular diseases and type 2 diabetes due to changes in lipid profiles and increased belly fat.

HOW GLP-1 MEDICATIONS WORK

In simple terms, GLP-1 medications work in four main ways: in the *brain* (how we think and feel about all things food), in the *gut* (how we digest and experience the actual eating of food), in *hormones* (how we use the food we eat within the complex metabolic and hormonal systems of our body), and in *reducing inflammation* (stress on the body).

1. **Brain**
    - Increase perception of satiety, improve motivation, adherence, and mental health, satisfaction with foods, change dietary preferences
    - Decrease anxiety around food, cravings, food noise; reduce interest in alcohol

2. **Gut**
    - Increase sensitivity and discomfort with high-fat or high-sugar foods
    - Decrease gastric emptying time so you feel fuller sooner on smaller portions

3. **Hormones**
    - Increase glucose uptake, improving ability to use carbohydrates for energy
    - Decrease insulin resistance, reducing ability to store excess calories as fat

4. **Inflammation**
    - Increase ability for macrophages to work, shifting these immune cells from promoting inflammation to helping reduce it
    - Decrease pro-inflammatory cytokines that cause inflammation and inhibit how inflammatory genes respond to triggers

How Do GLP-1 Medications Work?

GLP-1 medications work by mimicking one or two naturally produced hormones: glucagon-like peptide-1 (GLP-1) and gastric inhibitory polypeptide (GIP).

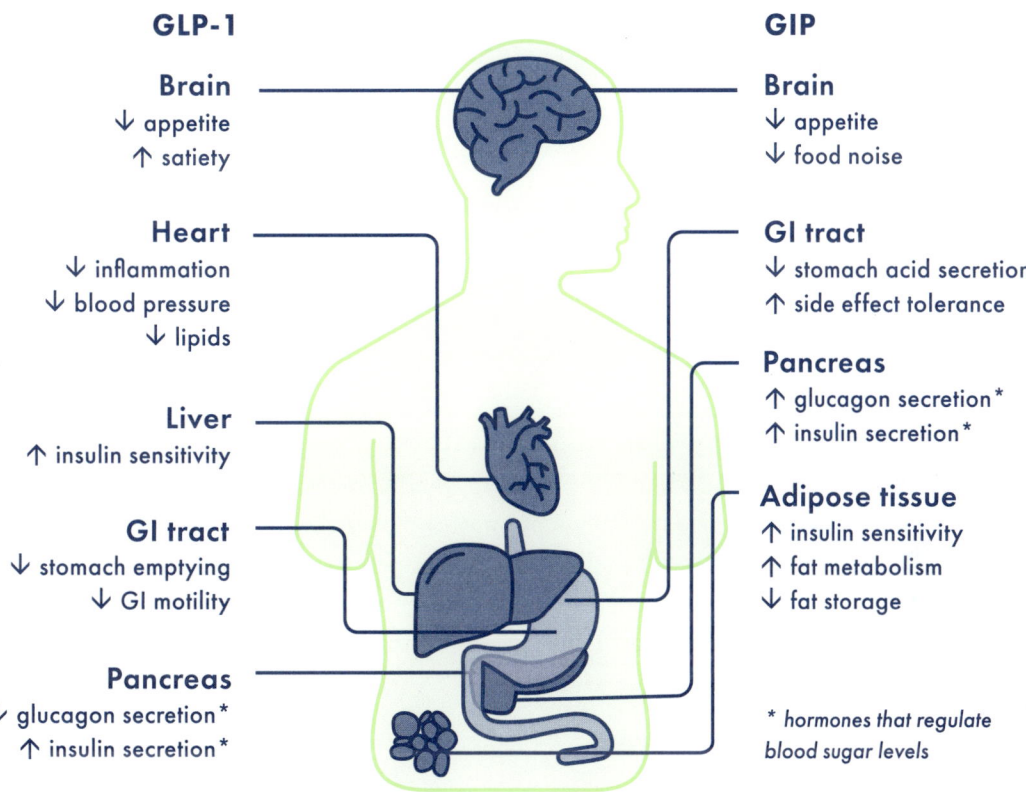

GLP-1

Brain
↓ appetite
↑ satiety

Heart
↓ inflammation
↓ blood pressure
↓ lipids

Liver
↑ insulin sensitivity

GI tract
↓ stomach emptying
↓ GI motility

Pancreas
↓ glucagon secretion*
↑ insulin secretion*

GIP

Brain
↓ appetite
↓ food noise

GI tract
↓ stomach acid secretion
↑ side effect tolerance

Pancreas
↑ glucagon secretion*
↑ insulin secretion*

Adipose tissue
↑ insulin sensitivity
↑ fat metabolism
↓ fat storage

* hormones that regulate blood sugar levels

Many GLP-1 drugs (like Ozempic and Wegovy) act by binding to GLP-1 receptors, resulting in the same effects of GLP-1 seen above.

However, some medications (like Mounjaro and Zepbound) are unique in that they bind to GLP-1 and GIP receptors, resulting in a combined effect.

MORE ON HORMONES

When someone uses a GLP-1 medication, certain hormones and their effects are impacted.

Amylin: GLP-1 medications increase the secretion of amylin, a hormone co-secreted with insulin. Amylin slows gastric emptying, reduces glucagon secretion after eating, and promotes satiety (feeling fuller sooner and longer), helping prevent rapid increases in blood glucose levels after meals. Limiting glucose spikes limits cravings, fat storage, and inflammation.

Ghrelin: Often referred to as the hunger hormone, ghrelin is produced primarily in the stomach and stimulates appetite, increases food intake, and promotes fat storage. Ghrelin levels typically rise before meals, stimulating hunger, and fall after eating. GLP-1 receptor agonists can lead to a reduction in ghrelin levels, which helps promote a feeling of fullness more quickly and sustains it longer, leading to lower overall calorie intake and weight loss.

Glucagon: GLP-1 medications decrease the secretion of glucagon from alpha cells in the pancreas. Glucagon usually increases blood sugar levels by stimulating glucose production in the liver. The liver produces and releases this glucose into the body when a person is under stress, fasting, or exercising. So, by suppressing glucagon, the liver can't release sugar and the person has better blood sugar control, regardless of what they eat.

Insulin: Insulin is produced by the beta cells of the pancreas and plays a crucial role in glucose metabolism by facilitating the uptake of glucose into cells, where it can be used for energy. Insulin also helps store excess glucose in the liver as glycogen and inhibits the breakdown of fat in adipose (fat) tissue. GLP-1 medications increase the secretion of insulin from the pancreas when blood glucose levels are high. This action is glucose-dependent, meaning it happens only after eating, so the risk of hypoglycemia (low blood sugar) is low.

Leptin: Leptin is produced primarily by adipose (fat) tissue and helps regulate energy balance by inhibiting hunger, which helps control food intake and body weight. Higher levels of leptin signal to the brain that the body has adequate energy stores, reducing appetite and promoting energy expenditure. While GLP-1 medications do not directly influence leptin levels, they do promote weight loss. It is this subsequent reduction in body fat that can lead to a decrease in circulating leptin levels because leptin production is proportional to fat mass. Weight loss achieved through the use of GLP-1 medications may also improve leptin sensitivity, meaning the body can now respond more effectively to leptin's signals, further aiding weight management.

Bonus Hormone: GIP

If you'll remember, while Wegovy and Ozempic (semaglutide) are single agonists of GLP-1, both Mounjaro and Zepbound (tirzepatide) are dual agonists, including both GLP-1 and gastric inhibitory polypeptide (GIP) incretin mimetics that work together for even greater improvements in blood sugar control and weight loss. GIP, also known as glucose-dependent insulinotropic polypeptide, is an incretin hormone that plays a significant role in the regulation of insulin secretion and glucose metabolism. GIP is produced by the K-cells in the upper parts of the small intestine (duodenum and proximal jejunum) in response to the ingestion of nutrients, particularly fats and carbohydrates. (GLP-1 is made in the stomach; GIP is made a little farther down.) GIP has been shown to promote the uptake and storage of lipids in adipose tissue where they belong and out of the blood where lipids are dangerous. It enhances the incorporation of fatty acids into triglycerides, playing a role in fat metabolism and storage. Some studies suggest that GIP may also have a role in bone density by influencing processes such as bone formation and resorption. Some experts suspect that GIP may play a role with the improvements in the GI side effects.

MORE ON INFLAMMATION

Although the primary benefits of GLP-1 medications are related to blood sugar regulation and weight loss, emerging research also suggests they also have anti-inflammatory effects. Almost every person I know who has taken these medications says something along the lines of "I don't know what it is, but I just *feel* so much better!"

We know that GLP-1 medications work by binding to the GLP-1 receptors, which are widely distributed, not only in the pancreas where it works its magic on insulin secretion but also in other tissues including immune cells. GLP-1 receptor activation on these immune cells is associated with a reduction in the levels of pro-inflammatory cytokines (proteins that make you feel awful). One of the most interesting ways GLP-1 medication works on immune system cells is what we see with macrophages. Macrophages are key immune cells that usually increase inflammation, but the GLP-1 receptor activation can shift macrophages from pro-inflammatory to anti-inflammatory, thereby reducing inflammation when stressed instead of increasing it!

Benefits of Reducing Inflammation

- Patients with type 2 diabetes often have elevated levels of inflammatory markers. The anti-inflammatory effects of GLP-1 medications can be particularly beneficial in managing diabetes-related complications such as neuropathy, kidney disease, and increased risk for stroke.

- Chronic inflammation is a major contributor to cardiovascular diseases. By reducing inflammation, GLP-1 medications can lower the risk of atherosclerosis and other cardiovascular conditions.

- Neuroinflammation is implicated in neurodegenerative diseases such as Alzheimer's and Parkinson's. GLP-1 receptor agonists have been shown to have neuroprotective effects, possibly by reducing inflammation in the brain.

- Inflammation is a known risk factor for the development and progression of certain cancers. There is some evidence to suggest that GLP-1 medications might have anticancer properties through their anti-inflammatory effects.

- Although still an area of active research, GLP-1 medications have shown promise in reducing inflammation associated with rheumatic and autoimmune conditions.

QUALIFICATIONS AND CONTRAINDICATIONS

Understanding who qualifies for these medications and who should avoid them can help ensure safe and effective treatments and outcomes. GLP-1 medications should be prescribed and monitored by a health care provider, typically an obesity medicine physician, endocrinologist, or primary care physician with experience in managing diabetes and obesity. Regular monitoring from health care providers, adherence to prescribed treatment plans, and monitoring for adverse effects are integral to successful therapy with GLP-1 medications. Adjustments to doses and long-term management plans are based on your unique progress and experience. Generally speaking, to qualify for GLP-1 medications, the FDA requires:

- Eligibility criteria for diabetes with an HbA1C, a lab value that shows your average blood glucose over the previous three months of ≥ 6.5 percent, and BMI > 27 kg/m^2.

- Eligibility criteria for obesity with a body mass Index (BMI) of ≥ 30 kg/m^2 (obese).

- You are also eligible with a BMI of ≥ 27 kg/m^2 (overweight) with at least one weight-related comorbidity, such as heart disease, hyperlipidemia, hypertension, or prediabetes (A1C > 5.7 percent).

Your insurance carrier may have additional requirements beyond the FDA guidelines. They argue that these are in place to control costs or inappropriate prescribing, but I see them as practicing medicine without a license and with obesity bias!

You may feel as though you are jumping through hoops to "prove" you've "tried" to lose weight before with traditional methods. For example, some plans may require step therapy (trying a lower-cost option first), nutrition counseling (three to six months of working with a doctor or dietitian before starting medication), proof of weight loss efforts (like receipts from Weight Watchers or Noom), or even a BMI > 35 or 40, depending on the plan. So, get your ducks in a row and be prepared to ask your provider to file appeals with supporting documentation.

There are, as with most pharmaceuticals, clinical reasons and contraindications for not taking GLP-1 medications, which include:

- **Active eating disorders:** GLP-1 medications can alter appetite and eating patterns. For individuals with a history of eating disorders (anorexia nervosa, bulimia nervosa), these changes might trigger unhealthy behaviors and contribute to a relapse. These medications might negatively influence individuals preoccupied with body weight and self-image, exacerbating their eating disorder symptoms. Common side effects of GLP-1 medications include nausea and vomiting, which can be particularly problematic for individuals with a history of bulimia nervosa, as it may precipitate or worsen purging behaviors. Care should be taken to ensure those with histories of eating disorders, common in people who have been living with obesity, are appropriately supported by mental health and nutrition care teams. Folks with binge-eating disorder, however, seem to benefit greatly from GLP-1 therapy.

- **Cost and insurance coverage:** The cost of these medications can be prohibitive and unaffordable for many, especially those without insurance coverage. (More on that later.)

- **Kidney problems:** GLP-1 medications require caution and are contraindicated in patients with severe renal impairment. The concern is primarily from the risk of dehydration after episodes of diarrhea or vomiting. Monitoring renal function is essential during treatment for anyone with a history of kidney disease. Good news is that research is showing that semaglutide may actually slow or reverse kidney disease, even for people on dialysis.

- **Multiple endocrine neoplasia syndrome type 2 (MEN 2):** Patients with MEN 2, a genetic condition that increases the risk of endocrine tumors, including medullary thyroid carcinoma, should avoid GLP-1 medications.

- **Pancreatitis:** A mild risk of pancreatitis is associated with GLP-1 medications; if you have a history of pancreatitis, avoid these drugs.

- **Patient preference:** Some patients may prefer other forms of diabetes management or weight loss interventions due to personal comfort or lifestyle considerations. Some may be averse to using injectables.

- **Personal or family history of medullary thyroid cancer (MTC):** GLP-1 medications have been linked to thyroid C-cell tumors in rodent studies.

- **Pregnancy and breastfeeding:** GLP-1 medications are not recommended for use while trying to conceive, during pregnancy, and while breastfeeding due to the lack of sufficient well-controlled studies in this population. The primary worry is inadequate nutrition, resulting in potential risks to the fetus or infant. GLP-1s also decrease the effectiveness of oral birth control and increase fertility, so plan accordingly!

- **Severe gastrointestinal disease history:** Pre-existing conditions such as gastroparesis can be exacerbated by GLP-1 medications, which may further slow gastric emptying and cause discomfort.

- **Severe gastrointestinal issues:** Common side effects include constipation, diarrhea, nausea, vomiting, and very low appetite. Although usually mild, these issues can negatively affect overall health and quality of life. If side effects are severe to the extent that they limit your ability to participate in usual activities, talk to your doctor.

- **Shortages:** Given the high demand and low overall supply, at times, these medications can end up in "shortage" and become difficult to find, resulting in gaps in treatment or the use of ineffective available doses.

- **Suicide history:** Although rare, some patients taking GLP-1 medications have reported mood changes, including increased anxiety and depression. For individuals with a history of suicide attempts, these potential side effects could contribute to a resurgence or worsening of suicidal ideation.

LET'S TALK ABOUT BMI

I get it; for some of us that BMI number brings up some big feelings and instant frustration. It's clearly imperfect, but perhaps not totally useless. Here are some pros, cons, and controversies to consider before putting too much weight (pun intended) into the number.

Pros of BMI

- **Simple and cost-effective:** BMI is easy to calculate using only height and weight, making it a low-cost tool for large-scale assessments. You can calculate it yourself: Divide your weight in kilograms by your height in meters and then divide that number by your height in meters again.

- **Widely used and standardized:** It provides a common metric across medical specialties and research.

- **Useful as a screening tool:** BMI helps identify individuals who **may** be at risk of obesity-related health problems.

Cons of BMI for Obesity

- **Does not distinguish between fat and muscle:** BMI cannot differentiate between fat and lean mass, leading to misclassification of muscular individuals as overweight or obese.

- **Ignores fat distribution:** BMI does not account for *where* excess weight is distributed; a person may have a "normal BMI" yet carry harmful visceral fat around their organs.

- **Not accurate for all populations:** The BMI is not universally applicable to different age groups, ethnicities, genders, or body types. Research suggests we are better protected from poor health at slightly higher BMIs as we enter advanced age.

Controversies of BMI for Obesity

- **Oversimplification:** BMI oversimplifies obesity and overall health by reducing it to a single number, ignoring factors such as genetics, lifestyle, and previous weight history.

- **Inappropriate for individual diagnosis:** BMI is best used as a population-level tool, using only BMI to determine individual diagnosis or treatment decisions can be misleading.

- **Cut-off points debate:** The BMI category cut-offs for normal (BMI of 19 to 24), overweight (BMI of 25 to 29.9), and obesity (BMI ≥ 30) are seen as arbitrary.

DEBUNKING COMMON MYTHS ABOUT GLP-1s

Okay, so you've seen the ways GLP-1 medications work and how and why they were created, let's dive into all the other "noise" you've probably heard.

GLP-1 medications have obviously been proven extremely effective and safe. They are FDA-approved and show results never before been seen by medication for diabetes and obesity. But, whether it's a distrust in science or some obesity bias at play, despite their growing popularity, misconceptions persist. I hope to debunk several common myths associated with GLP-1 medications and provide a more accurate representation of what we actually need to worry about.

Myth: GLP-1 medications are a quick fix or a jump-start for weight loss.

Reality: GLP-1 medications, such as Ozempic and Wegovy, are not magical. They don't work as intended in the absence of healthy nutrition and physical activity. They are also not intended to be taken short term. While we may be familiar with a "twenty-eight-day fix" or a "six-week cut," GLP-1 medications are meant to be part of a long-term treatment plan and work by targeting multiple pathways involved in appetite regulation and glucose control. Years of diets that never work show us that quick, temporary fixes do not address the underlying physiological and behavioral components of obesity.

Myth: GLP-1 medications cause stomach paralysis.

Reality: GLP-1 medications do slow gastric emptying, but this is not the same as stomach paralysis or the medical diagnosis of "gastroparesis." The slowing of gastric emptying helps reduce post-meal blood sugar spikes and promotes a feeling of fullness, aiding weight management. This effect is generally mild and transient. Although gastroparesis is a rare side effect experienced by some people who have taken GLP-1 medications, people with obesity and diabetes are already at increased risk for this condition. In other words, uncontrolled diabetes can cause gastroparesis. Unfortunately, even healthy people who are not on GLP-1s can experience bowel obstructions. Remember, correlation does not equal causation.

Myth: Using medications like Ozempic can cause "Ozempic face," a term for a sagging or gaunt facial appearance (also, Ozempic butt).

Reality: The term "Ozempic face" is not medically recognized. Any changes in facial appearance are likely due to significant weight loss rather than the medication itself. Rapid or substantial weight loss can sometimes lead to a loss of facial fat, which might change one's appearance. However, this is a consequence of weight loss, not specifically of the medication. It's a fact that we are conditioned to see faces that have more fat as youthful and healthy, but this does not mean a lean or more wrinkled appearance is problematic. The "Ozempic face" myth only serves to highlight the ways in which our culture tends to focus on appearance as more important than health or quality of life.

Myth: GLP-1 medications lead to muscle loss.

Reality: It's really hard to lose a significant amount of body weight without losing some muscle. Clinical studies have shown that while some muscle loss does occur with any method of weight loss, following a balanced diet rich in protein and incorporating resistance training can help preserve muscle mass during the process. Muscle is health-promoting and should be attended to, but there is no data to suggest that GLP-1 medications are specifically more muscle wasting than bariatric surgery or calorie restriction dieting.

Myth: GLP-1 medications are too new and so lack sufficient safety data.

Reality: GLP-1 medications have been studied extensively since the 1990s with the first medication, Byetta, coming to market in 2005. Mounjaro, Ozempic, Saxenda, Victoza, Wegovy, and Zepbound have undergone rigorous clinical trials and post-marketing surveillance, accumulating a substantial body of evidence supporting their safety and efficacy, and remain FDA approved. In 2024, the Wegovy SELECT trial published four-year data showing weight maintenance. Regulatory agencies such as the FDA continue to approve these medications for additional indications, such as cardiovascular disease, fatty liver, and sleep apnea, based on robust data. Not only are they safe for obesity and diabetes, they are also being explored for use in a variety of other conditions like substance use disorders and Alzheimer's disease.

Myth: GLP-1 medications are only for people with diabetes.

Reality: While GLP-1 medications were initially developed for type 2 diabetes management, their benefits extend to people with obesity and other metabolic disorders. The FDA has approved specific GLP-1 formulations for chronic weight management in individuals with or without diabetes. For the semaglutides, Ozempic (for diabetes) is the same medication as Wegovy (for obesity). For the tirzepatides, Mounjaro (for diabetes) is the same medication as Zepbound (for obesity). Any concerns regarding supply shortages are a failure of the manufacturer to meet demand, not patients seeking treatment for their FDA-approved indication.

Myth: GLP-1 medications can cause eating disorders.

Reality: There is no evidence to suggest that GLP-1 medications cause eating disorders. On the contrary, these medications help regulate appetite and improve eating behavior in individuals struggling with obesity or binge eating. I repeatedly hear from people taking these medications that they have never felt so at peace with food before. They no longer need to resort to restrictive or disordered food behaviors to manage their weight in a healthy way. People are able to practice eating intuitively, enjoy their favorite foods, and stop when they are full. People with active eating disorders should not start these medications as a means with which to achieve unhealthy or rapid weight loss; such concerns should be discussed with health care and mental health providers.

Myth: Taking GLP-1 medications is the easy way out for weight loss.

Reality: Using GLP-1 medications is not about seeking an easy solution but rather a medically appropriate one. Obesity is a complex chronic disease with genetic, environmental, and behavioral components. GLP-1 medications provide a scientifically validated option for managing obesity, demonstrating that addressing obesity requires more than just willpower. And really, why can't it be easier? It is clear that managing excess weight is hard enough without sufficient support. Suffering less is a good thing!

Myth: You must follow a strict diet and exercise plan when using GLP-1 medications.

Reality: While eating healthy, nutritious foods and physical activity are certainly encouraged to maximize the benefits of GLP-1 medications and maintain good health, they are not mandatory and don't need to be overly strict. These medications make it easier for individuals to adopt and maintain healthier lifestyle habits. Instead of having to micromanage, obsess, or tightly control every aspect of your nutrition, you can instead simply eat nutritious meals and lean into hunger and fullness cues for guidance. More later on these principles of nutritious eating in chapter 5, but "diet" it certainly is not.

Myth: You just need more willpower to lose weight rather than taking medication.

Reality: Obesity is influenced by numerous biological factors that go beyond individual willpower. Hormonal imbalances, genetics, and metabolic differences, in the context of environments, privileges, education, and access to foods, play significant roles. We have much less control over the way our body reacts to the world we live in than we'd like to believe. GLP-1 medications help address these complexities by regulating hunger hormones and improving metabolic health. Willpower and white-knuckling against food noise can only go so far and, eventually, the drive to eat gets so strong (because we get hungrier when we restrict or lose weight) it eventually cannot compete with our biology (those hormones that signal our brains and override our ability to make choices). GLP-1 medications enable adherence to our best intentions without the fight.

Myth: Natural alternatives work the same or are better and are safer than GLP-1 medications.

Reality: While natural remedies like dietary changes and physical activity are important, they might not be sufficient for everyone, especially those with significant metabolic challenges. Any natural supplements claiming to provide the same benefits as GLP-1 medications are a scam. GLP-1 medications are rigorously tested, standardized, and approved by regulatory bodies, providing a level of safety and efficacy that most natural alternatives cannot match. If berberine or probiotics produced the same results, big pharma would have cashed in on that decades ago.

CHAPTER 03

BUILDING A CARE TEAM AND NAVIGATING INSURANCE

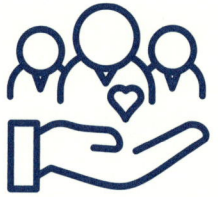

So, you've decided you're going to do this. You've examined the media landscape, talked to your family, and watched a few TikToks. You are excited about the hope that comes with knowing there may be some relief for your unmanageable appetite, something that can quiet the food noise and help you finally lose weight. So, where to start? Getting a prescription from a qualified provider—someone you trust, who is nonbiased against obesity as a disease, who understands the new science, and who can accurately assess whether you may qualify for treatment with GLP-1 medications—is a great first step. If you don't already have this resource in place, there are countless options. The ads are insistent—TV, social media, magazines—and it seems as though there are thousands of companies who can offer you a prescription online. I caution you to be a thoughtful consumer of your medical services. This isn't skin care or a hair product. This is anti-obesity medication with real risks to your health if not used under proper supervision.

HOW TO KNOW IF YOUR PROVIDER IS LEGIT?

- Do they have positive reviews and unpaid testimonials? Google, Reddit, and LinkedIn can be informative.

- Do they have the relevant licensures, education, and credentials?

- Do they hold malpractice insurance?

- Do they have experience? How many people have been successfully treated?

- Do they offer side effect management, nutrition, and fitness guidance and support?

- Can you access your care team with questions between visits or refills?

- Do they protect your privacy?

- Are fees and billing schedules transparent at sign-up?

- Do you feel seen, heard, and understood?

- Do you feel like they care about you as an individual?

BUILDING A CARE TEAM

Setting out to lose weight is best achieved with a comprehensive care team that's got your back every step of the way. The first step is to find providers who genuinely care about you and your goals. Start by asking your primary care doctor or other trusted health professionals for referrals. Look for health care pros who have specialized training in obesity medicine, endocrinology, or nutrition. The American Board of Obesity Medicine has a nifty search feature on their website to help you find a provider near you. We all deserve to work with providers who take the time to listen, show empathy, and practice shared decision-making. This partnership ensures your treatment plan feels right for you and matches your goals and lifestyle. Telehealth is incredibly convenient; you can speak with your provider from the comfort of your home, saving you time and the hassle of traveling. It's especially great for people who live in remote areas or have difficulty getting around. Scheduling frequent check-ins can improve outcomes, providing regular encouragement and adjustments as needed.

In-person care, on the other hand, allows for a more comprehensive evaluation. Your provider can do full physical examinations and detailed assessments. Building a strong face-to-face relationship can also enhance trust and communication. Access to drawing labs, treatments, and other services is another significant advantage. But, let's face it, traveling to appointments can be time-consuming, and fitting them into an already busy schedule can be tricky, especially if you have work or kids.

TALKING TO YOUR DOCTOR ABOUT STARTING A GLP-1

Although you've started reading up on the topic, preparing for your visit will also help! Being well-informed can help you articulate the benefits of GLP-1s as well as their potential side effects, allowing you to discuss them intelligently with your doctor. I recommend creating a list of your existing medications, dietary habits, exercise routines, and any complications or issues you've experienced due to your excess weight. Reflect on your personal health goals beyond just "weight loss" or appearance. Are you looking primarily to manage your blood sugar levels or reduce the risk of complications related to diabetes? Are you worried about your mobility? Clearly defining your goals will help your health care provider understand your motivations and expectations. You might say, "I've been working on controlling my blood sugar better and would also like to lose weight to improve my overall health. Do you think a GLP-1 medication could help with those goals?"

ASK QUESTIONS

Show up with questions. Even if you are already well-informed, speaking with your doctor is an opportunity for you to gauge your provider's comfort level and competency in prescribing this medication.

- How do GLP-1 medications work, and how do they compare to other weight loss medications?
- What are the potential side effects?
- Based on my health history, are there any reasons I shouldn't take GLP-1 medications?
- How do I administer a GLP-1 medication?

- What can I expect during treatment?
- How often can and should I follow up?
- What happens when I get to my goal weight?

Speak Openly

During your appointment, approach your doctor with open and honest dialogue. It's important to express any concerns or experiences that may be relevant to your treatment options. For example, you could say, "I'm concerned about my weight management and how it affects my diabetes. I've heard positive things about GLP-1 medications and would like to know your thoughts." If your doctor uses unfamiliar terms or concepts, ask for clarification. It's essential that you leave the appointment with a clear understanding of your treatment options.

Include Lifestyle

Discuss lifestyle changes as well; GLP-1 medications work best when paired with healthy habits. Share your current challenges by saying, "I've struggled to maintain a consistent exercise routine because of my busy schedule. Do you have any recommendations on how I can incorporate more activity into my daily life?"

Get a Second Opinion

Your physician may be hesitant to prescribe these medications, not because they are unsafe or because they don't work, but because they are so popular. Providers worry that patients will start these treatments without understanding the risks. If you are uncertain about your doctor's recommendations, seeking a second opinion is perfectly acceptable.

If, however, you and your doctor mutually decide that a GLP-1 medication is the right choice for you, it's important to schedule regular follow-ups to assess the medication's effectiveness, monitor any potential side effects, and adjust dosing as needed.

THE COST—IT'S NOT CHEAP

While GLP-1 medications are effective and helpful for most people, their benefits come at a significant monetary cost, raising questions about accessibility, long-term investment, and the overall impact on health care spending. In the absence of insurance coverage, the cost of GLP-1 medications varies widely, and many patients find the prices unaffordable. Ozempic, approved primarily for type 2 diabetes but also used off-label for weight loss, can cost $900 USD to $1,000 USD per month. Wegovy, which is approved specifically for weight management in adults with obesity, hovers between $1,300 USD and $1,500 USD per month. Mounjaro and Zepbound, which combine actions of GLP-1 and GIP (gastric inhibitory peptide), is similarly priced, ranging from $1,000 USD to $1,200 USD per month. These high retail prices represent a significant financial burden for many patients; however, some manufacturers provide coupons and patient savings programs to help.

Manufacturer coupons are a form of patient assistance that allows individuals to potentially lower their copay or out-of-pocket cost for prescribed medications. These programs, usually offered directly by pharmaceutical companies, may require patients to meet specific income or insurance criteria to be eligible. Those on government insurance plans, including military insurance, are often excluded from participation in these programs. For a patient who is prescribed Wegovy, the manufacturer's coupon may lower the monthly cost from over $1,300 USD to as little as $25 USD. Others, with the same coupon, may only save $250 USD if their insurance company isn't offering approval to some degree. While these programs offer much-needed financial relief for many, they are not a permanent solution and often lead only to short-term sustainability of treatment. Manufacturers can choose to end coupon programs at any time, leaving patients with suddenly elevated out-of-pocket costs.

When contemplating long-term treatment for obesity, individuals should thoughtfully consider all their options. One alternative to GLP-1 medications is bariatric surgery, which has its own set of costs. The upfront cost of bariatric surgery can range from $15,000 to $30,000, depending on the type of procedure and health care setting. Although the initial expense is considerable, many studies show that surgery can lead to significant weight loss and a decrease in obesity-related complications, potentially lowering overall health care costs in the long run. However, the lifetime costs of both GLP-1 medications and bariatric surgery warrant careful consideration. For individuals who may need to remain on GLP-1 medications for extended periods, the ongoing expenses can surpass the one-time cost of surgery. In many cases, a bariatric surgery is covered by an individual's insurance while GLP-1s are not.

The financial implications of obesity extend beyond medications and surgeries. Unmanaged obesity is linked to a variety of complications, including type 2 diabetes, heart disease, and joint problems. The lifetime costs associated with these complications can be staggering. Studies suggest that individuals with obesity may incur an additional $1,800 USD to $3,000 USD in health care costs per year related to untreated comorbidities. As we age, these costs can accumulate, leading to a more significant strain on both personal finances and the health care system.

Disparities in access to GLP-1 medications further complicate the landscape of obesity treatment. Marginalized communities often face barriers such as lack of insurance, underinsurance, and limited access to health care providers knowledgeable about these new therapies. These disparities can result in unequal access to both medications and the necessary support systems that assist with weight management. Additionally, cultural perceptions of obesity and varying health care priorities can influence how different populations engage with treatment options. Without concerted efforts to address these inequities, the potential benefits of GLP-1 medications may disproportionately favor wealthier individuals, exacerbating existing health disparities in obesity management across demographics.

NAVIGATING INSURANCE IN AMERICA IS A BITCH

Despite its complexities, the American health insurance system does offer significant benefits. Insurance plans generally provide comprehensive coverage, including preventive care, emergency services, and prescription drugs. Many plans also cover preventive services at no additional cost, which promotes early detection and treatment of health issues. Additionally, insurance networks provide access to a wide range of specialists and health care facilities, enhancing the quality and scope of care available.

KEY TERMS

If you have health insurance, navigating it is a complex endeavor, filled with numerous terms, options, and significant decisions that can profoundly affect your financial and physical well-being. At the heart of health insurance terminology are several key terms.

- **Premiums** are the amounts paid for health insurance plans, typically on a monthly basis. This cost ensures you have insurance coverage in place.

- **Deductibles** are the amount you must pay out of pocket for health care services before your insurance begins to cover the costs; plans with higher deductibles generally have lower premiums, and vice versa.

- **Copayment**, or copay, is a fixed amount paid for specific health care services at the time of service, such as doctor's visits or prescription medications.

- **Coinsurance** is the percentage of costs shared with your insurance company after meeting your deductible—if your coinsurance is 20 percent, you pay 20 percent of the costs and the insurance covers the remaining 80 percent.

- **Out-of-pocket maximum** is the limit on what you pay for covered services within a policy period, typically a year; once this limit is reached, the insurance company covers 100 percent of expenses for covered services.

- **Network** refers to the facilities, providers, and suppliers your health insurer has contracted with; in-network providers usually cost less than those out of network.

The system is not without its criticisms, though. As of 2023, it is estimated that about 28 million Americans, or about 8.6 percent of the population, are uninsured, highlighting a persistent issue within the health care system. The reasons for this lack of coverage are multifaceted.

- High costs—whether premiums, deductibles, or other out-of-pocket costs— are a significant issue, as US health care and insurance expenses are among the highest globally and can be prohibitive for many individuals and families, particularly those with lower incomes who do not qualify for Medicaid or other assistance programs.

- The system's complexity can be overwhelming, making it difficult for individuals to understand and navigate their options effectively.

- Coverage gaps in employer-sponsored insurance, especially for part-time or low-wage workers, contribute to the overall uninsured rate, with significant variations among plans; some necessary treatments may incur large out-of-pocket expenses.

- The fact that many Americans receive health insurance through their employers ties coverage to employment status, which can cause people to remain in problematic working environments for fear of being uninsured.

- Geographic disparities also play a role; some states have chosen not to expand Medicaid under the Affordable Care Act (ACA), a.k.a. Obamacare, leaving millions without access to affordable options.

PRIOR AUTHORIZATION

Prior authorizations are a frustrating step in the process, particularly when it comes to obtaining medications. Insurance companies often require health care providers to obtain approval before prescribing specific drugs or treatments to ensure they are medically necessary and appropriate for the patient's condition (*insert eyeroll here*). The prior authorization process usually starts when a doctor assesses a patient's needs and determines that a particular medication is the best therapeutic option. The health care provider must then submit a request to the insurance company, which includes documentation justifying the need for the medication based on clinical guidelines. The insurer reviews this information to determine if it meets their criteria for coverage. This process can sometimes lead to delays in treatment, as patients may have to wait for approval before they can access their prescribed medications. Additionally, it can create an administrative burden for health care providers, who must navigate the requirements and paperwork involved. Although prior authorizations are intended to control costs and ensure the appropriateness of care, they can also contribute to frustrations for both patients and providers. It is an intentional strategy of heath insurance companies to delay, deny, and depose your care in an effort to maximize shareholder profits.

PRACTICAL TIPS: NAVIGATING HEALTH INSURANCE TO OPTIMIZE BENEFITS

Navigating commercial health insurance can be complex, but with the right approach, you can optimize benefits and save money. Here are ten practical tips to help.

1. **Understand Your Needs**

   Assess your health needs and those of your family. Consider factors like ongoing treatments, frequency of doctor visits, and any anticipated medical services. Consider that even if your medication isn't fully covered, a plan that covers other needs may well save you money in the long run.

2. **Compare Plans**

   Use comparison tools or websites to evaluate plans. Compare premiums, deductibles, copayments, and out-of-pocket maximums to find the best fit. Your employer should offer assistance in fully understanding your options before making selections.

3. **Review Provider Networks**

   Determine whether your preferred doctors and specialists are in network for the plans you're considering. Out-of-network care can significantly increase your costs.

4. **Find and Use Available Preventive Services**

   Many plans cover preventive services at no cost. Utilize annual checkups, vaccinations, and screenings to catch health issues early without additional costs.

5. **Understand Prescription Drug Coverage**

   Review the plan's formulary (list of covered drugs) and tier levels. Choose plans that provide better coverage for your medications to reduce costs.

6. **Maximize Health Savings Accounts (HSAs) or Flexible Spending Accounts (FSAs)**

   If eligible, contribute to HSAs or FSAs. These accounts allow you to use pre-tax dollars for qualified medical expenses, effectively lowering your overall costs.

7. **Utilize Telehealth Services**

   Many plans now offer telehealth options, which can be a cost-effective way to consult with health care providers without the expense of in-person visits.

8. **Know Your Rights**

   Familiarize yourself with the specifics of your plan, including what is covered, exclusions, and your appeal rights. This knowledge can help you advocate for your benefits.

9. **Keep Track of Medical Expenses**

   Maintain records of all medical expenses, receipts, and communications with your insurance provider. This can help in case of disputes and for tax deductions.

10. **Review Annually**

    Health needs and plans change. Review your options every year during open enrollment to ensure you have the most cost-effective plan that meets your needs.

SEEK EMPLOYER ASSISTANCE

Working with your employer to improve health insurance coverage or seek special exceptions for specialty medications can be a crucial step in accessing necessary medical care. The first step in this process is establishing open communication with your employer's human resources (HR) department or benefits coordinator. This dialogue can provide invaluable insight into the plan's structure and the potential for enhancements. In some cases, employers may have the ability to adjust plan features, such as increasing coverage limits or providing access to different medication tiers, especially if there is documented evidence of how these changes would benefit overall employee health and productivity. Let's be real here though, as I do not wish to provide false hope: You're unlikely to see immediate movement from

HR for individual cases; however, continued pressure from you—and others—could eventually move the needle.

If you are facing challenges accessing specialty medications, gather your pertinent medical information, including your doctor's recommendations and any prior authorization requests submitted to the insurance company. Presenting this information during your discussions with your employer's HR representative can offer a strong case supporting your need for special exceptions. In some situations, employers can exert some influence over insurance carriers, particularly if they can demonstrate that specific medications are critical for the health and well-being of employees. Employers often have the power to initiate appeals for coverage denials or work with the insurance provider to obtain necessary authorizations more swiftly.

Your employer may also offer health advocacy programs that can assist employees in navigating the complexities of insurance claims and exceptions. Persistence is key. If initial discussions do not yield immediate results, consider following up with additional documentation from your health care provider or building a community and collecting testimonials from other employees experiencing similar issues. Building a coalition of employees who face similar challenges can strengthen your case and demonstrate to your employer the widespread need for change.

It is also beneficial to stay informed about your rights under the Affordable Care Act, which may provide additional avenues for appealing coverage decisions or fighting against excessive out-of-pocket costs for medically necessary treatments. By actively participating in discussions with your employer and leveraging advocacy resources, you can work toward meaningful improvements to your health insurance coverage that facilitate access to the medications and care you need.

UNINSURED OR NOT TRADITIONALLY EMPLOYED

Funding health care when uninsured, unemployed, or working as a freelancer can be challenging, especially when it comes to managing costs. It may be worthwhile to explore the ACA marketplaces that offer private insurance plans. While unlikely to outright cover the full cost of GLP-1 therapy, having insurance is a common requirement to use the pharmaceutical company's discount coupons.

When brand-name GLP-1 weight loss medications are unavailable or prohibitively expensive, compounded versions can be a more affordable option. However, it's important to ensure that the compounding pharmacy is reputable and follows safety regulations, as the quality of compounded medications can vary. (We will discuss compounds in more detail in chapter 4.)

If you need medical supervision while using GLP-1 medications, consider visiting a sliding scale clinic or community health center. These facilities offer reduced-cost health care services based on your income.

Health care sharing programs are another option for those without traditional insurance. These programs allow members to pool their funds and share in covering health care costs.

HOLISTIC APPROACH TO OBESITY MANAGEMENT

I think it's a mistake to focus only on weight when treating obesity. It's not just about dropping pounds; it's about improving your overall health and well-being. Your mindset, nutrition, and fitness habits can all improve to support better health even if the scale doesn't move.

Behavioral therapies and mental health counseling can help you identify emotional triggers that lead to overeating, develop a healthier relationship with food, and manage stress in more constructive ways. Nutrition plans should be tailored to your tastes, lifestyle, and cultural background, making it easier for you to stick with it. Exercise plans should be enjoyable and sustainable, encouraging you to stay active and remain consistent. Additionally, having a solid support system—whether from family, friends, or support groups—can provide much-needed encouragement and motivation to keep going.

It's also crucial to remember that not all health problems can be solved by weight loss alone. Health metrics like blood pressure, blood sugar levels, and cholesterol levels are vital indicators of your overall well-being. You might be in great health despite not losing much weight; conversely, you could lose weight and still face health issues. So, it's important to focus on overall wellness, not just the number on the scale. This balanced approach helps you appreciate the various aspects of being healthy and encourages you to make sustainable changes.

Regular physicals and screenings are also important for effective obesity management. These checkups can identify potential health issues early, allowing for timely interventions. Regular screenings should include blood pressure checks to monitor your cardiovascular health, blood tests to track glucose, cholesterol levels, and liver function, and body measurements like BMI, waist circumference, and body fat percentage. Mental health evaluations are also crucial because addressing underlying issues such as depression or anxiety can affect your success in managing obesity. Having a comprehensive understanding of your health can help you and your provider collaboratively plan next steps.

Obesity is commonly correlated with increased cancer risks. Understanding when to start recommended cancer screenings can make a difference in early detection and successful treatment. Most health care guidelines recommend that individuals begin routine screenings at different ages, depending on the type of cancer being screened for. It's always best to consult with your health care provider to create a personalized screening schedule based on your individual risk factors and family history. By staying proactive and adhering to these recommended timelines, you can improve your chances of identifying potential issues early when they are most treatable.

CANCER SCREENING GUIDELINES

- Regular skin checks for skin cancer are recommended annually starting in the twenties, or earlier for those at a higher risk.

- Cervical cancer screenings, such as Pap smears, typically begin at age twenty-one, or within three years of becoming sexually active.

- Women should begin mammogram screenings for breast cancer at age forty, or earlier if they have a family history of the disease.

- Both men and women are advised to start colorectal cancer screenings at age forty-five.

- Prostate cancer screenings for men generally begin at age fifty, but those with a higher risk, such as African American men or people with a family history, should consider starting earlier.

- Lung cancer screenings, typically involving a low-dose CT scan, are advised for those aged fifty to eighty with a significant smoking history.

INCLUDE A REGISTERED DIETITIAN ON YOUR TEAM

A registered dietitian is a health care professional who specialize in food and nutrition, using their expertise to help individuals develop healthy eating habits, manage chronic conditions, and achieve sustainable weight management. Personalized nutritional guidance from a registered dietitian has proven to be a valuable resource to people trying to lose weight.

A REGISTERED DIETITIAN'S ROLE ON YOUR CARE TEAM

Registered dietitians (RDs) provide tailored nutrition plans that consider an individual's medical history, lifestyle, and personal preferences. This personalized approach increases the likelihood of enjoyment and adherence to the plan and long-term success. For example, RDs can create structured plans for individuals with prescriptive nutrition goals (like calories, grams of protein or fiber, including or excluding specific foods) that align with cultural food preferences and address specific health conditions such as diabetes, heart disease, and hypertension.

RDs rely on the latest scientific research to provide evidence-based nutrition recommendations. Their expertise ensures that individuals receive accurate, safe, and effective advice. This is particularly important given the prevalence of misinformation and fad diets that can harm rather than help. Addressing obesity often involves behavioral changes that can be challenging to maintain. RDs employ counseling techniques, like motivational interviewing, to support individuals when making sustainable lifestyle changes. This can include strategies for mindful eating, managing emotional eating, and setting realistic, achievable goals. Nutritional therapy provided by RDs has been shown to improve outcomes for various chronic conditions. Beyond disease management, by promoting healthy eating patterns and physical activity, RDs help individuals maintain a healthy weight, reduce the risk of chronic diseases, and improve overall well-being.

HOW TO FIND A DIETITIAN IN YOUR COMMUNITY

Finding a registered dietitian (RD) in your community or online can be a straightforward process, especially if you know where to look. Start by checking reputable sources such as the Academy of Nutrition and Dietetics website, where you can use their "Find a Nutrition Expert" tool. This allows you to search for RDs based on your location, specific dietary needs, and areas of expertise. You can also call your insurance company or ask your primary care physician for a referral, as they often work closely with a network of dietitians and can recommend someone who fits your requirements.

Local health clinics, hospitals, and community centers frequently employ dietitians, so exploring these options can lead you to qualified professionals nearby. Additionally, some gyms and wellness centers offer nutrition counseling services. Look for those that promote registered dietitians for their specific training and credentials rather than generic nutritionists.

If you prefer online consultations, many dietitians now offer virtual services. When you find potential candidates, review their credentials, areas of specialization, and client testimonials to ensure they align with your health goals. Reaching out for an initial consultation can help you assess their approach and whether it fits your needs, making it easier to embark on your journey toward better nutrition.

WHAT TO EXPECT IN A REGISTERED DIETITIAN APPOINTMENT

Meeting with a registered dietitian can be a little scary, especially if you don't know what to expect. Often, people worry they will be judged for their lifestyle or food behaviors or preferences. It's not a dietitian's job to judge or tell you what to do! Rather, they'll guide you through a conversation that explores options and then build a plan that brings you happiness and health.

Your first session is primarily about building a connection. Expect to spend a bit of time discussing your health history, lifestyle, and specific nutrition goals. You should feel welcome, comfortable, and heard.

Nutrition counseling is not just about what to eat. It's a holistic approach to achieving your personal goals and includes discussing the emotional and social aspects of eating and exploring how your mindset and environment can influence your choices. Together with the RD, you'll brainstorm strategies to create a balanced, enjoyable nutrition plan that aligns with your goals and is realistic for your life. This may include meal planning tips, snack ideas, or recommendations for incorporating more fruits and vegetables into your meals. The goal is to make these changes feel achievable and realistic, not overwhelming.

Nutrition counseling is a journey, not a one-time event. During follow-up sessions, you'll review progress, celebrate successes, and address any challenges.

REGISTERED DIETITIAN VS. NUTRITIONIST

While the two seem similar, there are important differences in terms of education, training, and professional requirements.

Registered Dietitian

A registered dietitian (RD), also known as a registered dietitian nutritionist (RDN), is qualified to provide medical nutrition therapy, develop personalized diet plans, and work in various settings such as hospitals, schools, and private practices. To achieve this credential, RDs must first earn at least a bachelor's degree in dietetics, nutrition, food science or a related field from an accredited program, such as the Accreditation Council for Education in Nutrition and Dietetics (ACEND).

Beyond academic coursework, an RD must complete a supervised ACEND-accredited practice program (internship), typically unpaid and about six to twelve months long, and then successfully complete a national examination administered by the Commission on Dietetic Registration (CDR).

To maintain registration, RDs engage in continuing professional education throughout their careers. Many states also have additional licensure requirements and can revoke a dietitian's credentials if the dietitian causes harm.

Nutritionist

The term "nutritionist" covers a broader and less standardized range of qualifications. Nutritionists should provide only general nutrition advice. You may see nutritionists working in community health, wellness, or education settings.

Some nutritionists hold degrees in nutrition, dietetics, public health, or related fields, but the requirements to become a nutritionist are not as clearly defined as they are for RDs. Certain states may require nutritionists to obtain certification and pass an exam, but many do not. In many places, the term "nutritionist" is not legally regulated, allowing individuals to use the title without any formal training or education.

It's perfectly normal to have setbacks, and your RD can help you navigate those hurdles without shame or guilt, adjusting your plan as needed to serve you well.

Throughout the process, I encourage you to ask questions and share any concerns. This is a two-way street, and your feedback is invaluable. Expressing what feels good and what doesn't allows your RD to tailor sessions to your needs. Nutrition counseling isn't about perfection; it's about progress. Together, you'll work to develop healthy habits that fit your life, ensuring a sustainable approach to well-being that can last a lifetime.

WORKING WITH YOUR DIETITIAN

If you're already working with a dietitian but are unsure of what to discuss in your sessions, consider some of these topics that can be very useful in long-term maintenance (on GLP-1s or not).

- Role of processed foods vs. whole foods (Maybe not as black and white as you think!)

- Nutrition quality and nutrients of concern (Am I getting all essential vitamins from foods or are supplements warranted?)

- Portion sizes (Maybe it's time to start adding food!)

- Food shopping, label reading (Understanding these skills can help you eat the way you know you want to.)

- Mindfulness practices, hunger/fullness cues (Your hunger cues are probably changing; it's likely this will be a lifelong journey of adjustments.)

- Gut health, microbiome, fiber targets (Healthy poops, anyone?)

- Reducing saturated fats, adding healthy fats (Nutrition is about more than just weight; good fats make for happy brains and hearts!)

- Alcohol and sugar (There's a fine line between a balanced and livable approach and consuming these potentially harmful foods in excess.)

- Regularity of eating patterns (No more skipping meals, avoiding the bingeing/restricting trap.)

- Managing sleep and stress (This affects insulin resistance and food choices, and life sometimes gets in the way. Am I controlling what I can?)

- Effects of hormone changes, pregnancy, and menopause (Our bodies change and may not behave in the same ways over time. Are you prepared to adjust?)

- Family changes, like divorce, new relationships, death of parents, job change, move (Life sucks sometimes, but our health and nutrition can still be a priority.)

- Dining out, traveling, vacations (Research shows these are the most common pitfalls to adhering consistently to a healthful nutrition plan.)

- Cooking skills and recipe modification (Skills require practice and continuous learning—enjoy the process!)

While, of course, I would love to work with each and every one of you as your personal dietitian, there simply are not enough hours in the day! And so here we are with this book! In the following chapters, I share with you all of my best advice, tips, and skills to support your GLP-1 journey to be the most nutritious, enjoyable, and healthy experience possible—for both your body and mind!

CHAPTER 04

GETTING STARTED ON A GLP-1

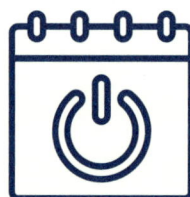

Getting started on your medication can be a little nerve-racking. You're learning so much new information and new skills and feeling so much hope and excitement! You might be nervous too—I know I was! Knowing what lies ahead (and what's important) at this stage in your journey is key to feeling confident and capable.

In this chapter we are going to talk about what to expect in those critical first few weeks: what to expect with side effects, how to approach your nutrition (in the beginning), how much weight you should be losing, and how to navigate potential issues at the pharmacy. Remember, this isn't a quick fix—we're in this for the long haul. Change can be hard, and it's more than okay if these first few weeks (or months) feel tricky. Hang in there, I got you.

PICKING UP YOUR PRESCRIPTION

I'm so excited for you! Your clinician has written your prescription! You've downloaded the manufacturer coupon! Ideally, your insurance approved the prior authorization and is covering some of the medication's cost (after you meet your deductible, of course). Or you've found room in your budget to treat your obesity with a GLP-1 medication. Hopefully, your medication is in stock, or at least on order, and will arrive at your pharmacy soon! Be kind to and patient with your pharmacy team—GLP-1 medications can sometime be tricky to process through insurance; just because you know your prior authorization was approved doesn't mean they know it yet. And running a manufacturer coupon properly is also, frankly, a pain in the ass! Shortages and delays are common with these medications, but hang in there, you'll get started soon.

PROPER STORAGE

Storing GLP-1 medications properly is critical to maintaining their efficacy and safety. These medications typically require refrigeration at temperatures between 36°F and 46°F (2°C and 8°C) until they are used. Once a GLP-1 medication is taken out of the refrigerator, it can generally be kept at room temperature, between 59°F and 86°F (15°C and 30°C), for a limited period as specified by the manufacturer—often 21 to 28 days. It's essential to protect the medication from excessive heat, direct sunlight, and freezing conditions, as these can degrade the active ingredients, rendering the medication ineffective. Refer to the specific storage guidelines

PRO TIP

Let the pen sit at room temperature for about 30 minutes before injecting to help prevent a stinging or burning sensation on administration. The needle is so fine you may not even feel the prick. A little bubble of fluid on your skin is normal. And a small bruise is also a possibility.

provided with the medication, and consult a health care provider if you have any concerns or uncertainties about storage conditions.

GIVING THE FIRST INJECTION

Once you get your medication home, the first major decision is whether it will live in the cheese drawer or the refrigerator door. It's normal to feel nervous, to doubt your decision, to even think about giving "diet and exercise alone" one last hurrah. But eventually, you open the box, read the package insert, maybe even watch a YouTube video to learn how to use the injector. Every medication has a slightly different pen mechanism:

- For Mounjaro and Zepbound, you must wait for the double click.
- The Wegovy pen has a yellow bar that needs to go all the way to the end.
- The Ozempic math with the clicks, whose idea was that?

Follow your prescriptions instructions carefully and set the pen to the correct dose before injecting. With practice, you will feel more comfortable. You may question whether you did it right, but I believe in you. You'll figure it out.

GUIDELINES AND CONSIDERATIONS FOR ADMINISTERING GLP-1s

While I encourage you to read the fine print in your package insert for your particular medication, I highlight here some important bits of information you should keep in mind to ensure your safety.

Consistency of Absorption and Injection Site Rotation

Variability in fat distribution and skin thickness across different injection sites (abdomen, buttocks, upper arm, upper thigh) can lead to differences in the consistency of drug absorption. The abdomen tends to offer more uniformity, whereas the thigh may present greater variability in how quickly the drug is absorbed. It is very normal to feel like you prefer one site over another, but it is important to rotate injection sites to maintain consistent absorption rates and reduce skin complications.

Recommended Injection Sites

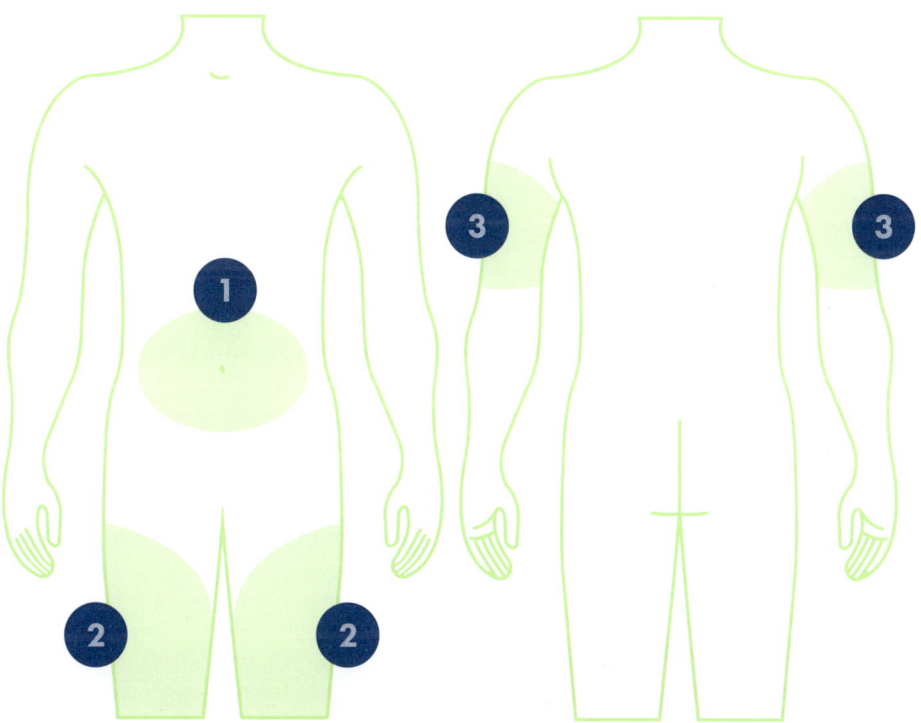

DOES INJECTION SITE REALLY MATTER?

There is some debate as to whether your injection site matters. The clinical research says that the abdomen, thigh, or back of the upper arm are all acceptable areas with subcutaneous fat in which the medication can be administered. The differences in amount of weight lost and degree of side effects' severity were not clinically significant from one site to the other. However, on an individual level, its normal to feel a difference. Some people experience more appetite suppression or fewer side effects from a particular site. Try them all to see whether you notice a difference and then do what works for you.

TO SHARE OR NOT TO SHARE?

When I was first prescribed my GLP-1 medication, I didn't tell a soul. "What will people think? I'm a freaking dietitian!" The internalized bias and shame held strong. I spent four more weeks counting macros and increasing my exercise before I finally took that first shot.

On day one, only my husband and Dr. Spencer knew. That was until the next morning when I could no longer contain my excitement after realizing I had forgotten to stop for coffee on my hour-long commute. I had gotten to work without even thinking about food! So, I figured I needed to eat something. In the cafeteria, the chef was pouring hot fresh tots into the buffet—and I felt instantly *turned off*. *What the hell is happening to me?*

I did, however, feel obligated to share my decision with my social media audience, many of whom had followed me for years. I explained the decision, took questions, and told the story about not thinking about food all day. The absolute relief. The quieting of the food noise. How not overeating for the first time in my life felt effortless. The outpouring of support was overwhelming. Of course, some folks didn't believe me—until they started their own journeys. At the time, no one was talking about this. It was so new that the news media had barely even heard of Ozempic. I became an early resource and, well, here we are now.

Deciding whether to share your journey is your decision alone. You have no obligation to disclose your personal medical treatment with others. However, I do think it's important to tell someone you trust—a spouse, a friend, a family member. If there is someone you share a lot of meals with, they will notice. The power of a support network in weight loss success and long-term maintenance is clear. You may even be pleasantly surprised when friends and family disclose their GLP-1 journey once you reveal yours.

Some patients may experience localized skin reactions, such as redness, swelling, or itching. Please report these to your health care provider. Over-the-counter hydrocortisone or antihistamine creams can be applied to reduce itching and inflammation.

Proper Injection Technique

Always clean the injection site with an alcohol swab before administering the medication to prevent infection and ensure that the correct needle size and length are used. Using a shorter needle can help reduce tissue trauma. If using an Ozempic or Saxenda pen, make sure your needles are compatible. Pinching the skin slightly can help avoid injecting into the muscle.

Administer the injection at the correct angle (usually 90 degrees) and depth to ensure it goes into the subcutaneous tissue, not deeper.

Managing a Pen Malfunction

Encountering a misfire or malfunctioning pen when administering a GLP-1 medication can be frustrating, but it's important to handle the situation correctly to ensure your safety and continued treatment. If the pen fails, do not attempt to dismantle it or troubleshoot beyond basic checks, like ensuring the needle is attached securely and there are no visible clogs or damages. Dispose of the malfunctioning pen in a sharps container to prevent accidental needle sticks.

Check in with your provider and follow their instructions for managing missed or partial doses. Depending on your dose, side effect history, and treatment goals, you may be instructed to take your next dose or hold off until the following week. Then, notify your pharmacist about the issue; they can provide guidance on next steps, including how to obtain a replacement pen. Most manufacturers also have customer support lines you can call for assistance and potential replacement options.

Using a Sharps Container

Always dispose of the used pen or needles in a sharps container. You can purchase these containers at pharmacies, medical supply stores, or online. Some health care providers may also offer them at no cost.

To prevent accidental needle sticks, never attempt to overfill the container. To exchange or dispose of a full sharps container, follow your local community guidelines. Many communities offer designated drop-off locations, including pharmacies, hospitals, or public health departments. Some areas also offer mail-back programs or household hazardous waste collection services. And note: These medical devices contain needles that can pose a risk of injury and potential transmission of blood-borne diseases to sanitation workers if simply thrown in the trash.

WHAT TO EXPECT THE FIRST FEW WEEKS

In the first several weeks on the starting doses of your medication, you may not feel *that* different. Ideally, you'll find some relief from an abnormally big appetite, have very few, if any, side effects, but still feel hungry at meal times. **Let me be clear: You still very much need to eat.**

You may have some side effects initially that make eating more challenging, but they typically resolve with time. It is a common misconception that GLP-1 medication is just to help you restrict food or diet or skip meals or never be hungry. The actual goal is for you to feel fuller and more satisfied on healthy portions of balanced meals; to make your big appetite a normal appetite; and to make it from one meal to the next meal without feeling drawn to any food that may cross your path. Because you ate your nutritious breakfast and are full is why you can say no to the baked goods a coworker brings to the break room every day. It's very normal for some to say, *I'm not sure if my medication is working*, then find themselves eating smaller portions of their usual foods, finding it easier to make the nutritious choices, and noticing a few pounds lost on the scale—without having to overthink it.

But it is also normal to not see this result on the scale or effect on the appetite right away. Some research suggests that about 30 percent of people who start GLP-1 medications don't see much benefit or weight loss for the first twelve weeks until they titrate up their dose to a more effective level, but often discontinue their treatment too soon as a result.

SAFE RATES OF WEIGHT LOSS

It's important to be realistic and safe with your weight loss goals. Slow and steady weight loss is recommended to preserve lean muscle mass, feel your best, and improve the chance of long-term maintenance. If you're losing weight too quickly, you aren't eating enough. A goal of around 1 percent weight loss per week is plenty. This means if you start your journey at 300 pounds (136 kg) and are losing more than 3 pounds (1.4 kg) per week, I'm worried about you.

The GLP-1 medications, although slightly different from each other, when combined with good nutrition and fitness, typically result in a 20 percent total body weight loss over the course of a year. So, if starting at 300 pounds (136 kg); you can realistically expect to lose about 60 pounds (27 kg). Some may lose more and some may lose less. Please remember, weight loss is not the only goal of effective obesity treatment. The numerous nonscale measure of progress—metabolic health improvements, reduced diabetes risk, improvement in hypertension and heart disease, improved kidney health, improvements in sleep apnea symptoms, reduced anxiety around food, improved energy, improved mobility, reduced inflammation—all seem to occur independent of weight lost.

LEARNING NEW HUNGER AND FULLNESS CUES

It's not uncommon to hear patients on GLP-1 medications say something like, "I'm not really sure when I'm hungry anymore." Because of this, it's easy to fall into the unrecommended pitfall of skipping meals. When you've lived your whole life with an insatiable appetite, it's hard to know what hungry even means anymore. Sometimes, we look to our bellies to rumble or to suddenly be thinking about food—but now on a GLP-1 medication, this rarely occurs. Your new hunger cues may be more subtle than those past. You may notice a slight headache, a dip in energy, or a change in mood. Instead of "I'm so hungry I need to eat NOW," it's more like "Oh, it's mealtime, I guess I should eat." Instead of, "OMG I really want this particular food," you think, "Something fresh sounds nice; let's see what there is." When your hunger comes on more slowly, it is more manageable. You have time now to make an intentional choice. The choice that will help your body feel its best, satisfy your preferences, keep you full for several hours, and meet your nutrition goals.

Fullness will feel different too. At first, it may be overwhelming or uncomfortable, but this gets better with time. Fullness may look like unintentionally putting your fork down before you've cleaned your plate or not finishing foods that just weren't that great. Sometimes, a meal will be so yummy you want to finish it—and you will—and maybe soon after reflect back and say, "I'm SO full; maybe I didn't need those last few bites." Fullness may not be a mental desire to stop eating; it might be physical, like a little hiccup or burp, or, hopefully rarely, nausea or reflux.

HUNGER AND FULLNESS SCALE

A guide to help you connect with your body to learn when and how much to eat. Eating three balanced meals per day at regular intervals can help you live comfortably between a 3 and 8.

OVERLY FULL

1 Extremely full, overly stuffed, just completed a massive meal with larger than normal portions, perhaps some regret

2 Uncomfortably full, a few bites too many, will be full for a while longer than usual

3 Comfortably full, no desire to eat more, happily satisfied, feels good

COMFORTABLE TIME TO STOP EATING

4 Could eat more but could stop, not sure, depends if I really love it

5 Neutral, not hungry, not full, indifferent, content, not really thinking about food

6 Could eat something small but also could wait, not sure, depends on if I really love it

NORMAL EATING RANGE

7 Could use a snack, but it's not urgent, depends how long until next meal or if I need fuel for activity

8 Could eat a full meal, getting low on energy, stomach feels empty, happy to eat something I like

9 Ravenous, getting hangry, moody, a little fatigue, need to eat ASAP, might overeat

OVERLY HUNGRY

10 Extremely hungry, exhausted, waited way too long, starving

Slowing down and paying attention while you eat will help. As you learn your new hunger and fullness cues, you will also learn how much to put on your plate.

NUTRITION IN THE FIRST FEW WEEKS

My most important tip when starting a GLP-1 medication is **don't overdiet.** Seriously, hear me out. Here's the thing about these medicines that is truly just so cool: Instead of restricting or eliminating certain foods, eating perfectly (as if there is such a thing), or weighing and measuring every bite, lick, or taste, you can just eat three balanced meals that don't make you feel unwell and move on with your life. The first few weeks on the medication are intended to get your body acclimated, to learn how you will feel after eating a variety of foods and figure out what will work for you. The first few weeks are *not* for weight loss, although weight loss will probably occur. Remember, it is normal, though, for some people to see little or no weight loss at their starting doses, so please, don't freak out.

In the first few weeks on GLP-1 medications, your job is to do just two things:

1. **Eat and Drink Enough**

    Eating and hydrating enough will look a little different for everyone because we all have different bodies, ages, sex assigned at birth, activity levels, and medical conditions. But generally speaking, you'll just want to avoid very large meals in those first few weeks.

    When it comes to food, plan to eat at least three meals per day. **A meal contains a healthy serving of lean protein (at least a 4-ounce [155 g by weight] serving size that provides 20 to 30 grams of protein), a fiber-full starchy carbohydrate (like grains, potatoes, or whole wheat pasta), and a plant (fruit or vegetable).** It is that simple. There will be time in the coming months to optimize your nutrition, and I dig into the details and nuances of my nutrition approach in future chapters, but for now, there's no need to rush the process. Eat enough food to have energy.

    It's also important to be aware that hydration can fall behind. In the same way your appetite is reduced, your thirst is reduced. Fill your favorite cup with a zero-calorie beverage and keep sipping. Most people need about

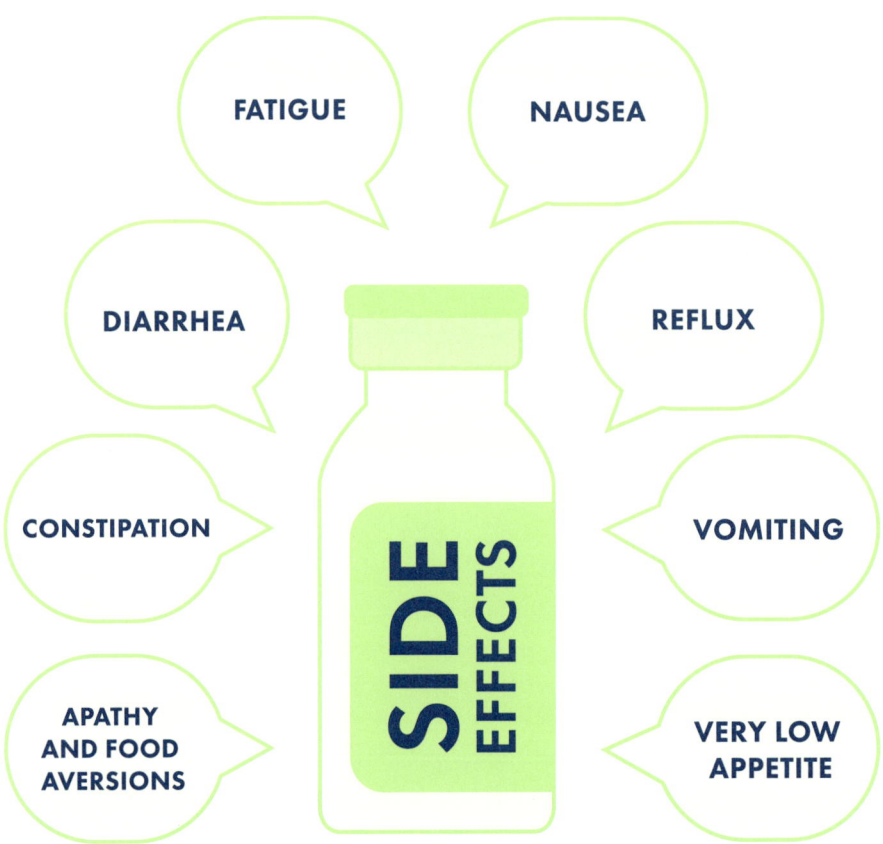

FATIGUE

NAUSEA

DIARRHEA

REFLUX

CONSTIPATION

VOMITING

SIDE EFFECTS

APATHY AND FOOD AVERSIONS

VERY LOW APPETITE

72 fluid ounces (2.1 L) per day, more or less depending on climate and activity. Look for light-colored urine and moist eyes, mouth, and skin.

2. **Manage Side Effects**

Successfully eating and drinking enough in the first few weeks of starting a GLP-1 medicine is most complicated by the potential for side effects. Obesity medicine specialists are clear that most side effects for most people on these medicines should be mild in severity, short-lived in duration, and easily managed with over-the-counter or nutrition interventions. As you are under the care of a prescriber, I encourage you to reach out to them to keep them informed and help you manage side effects. There are some tips, though, to help you feel informed and empowered to self-manage side effects as best you can in real time.

Apathy toward food and food aversions. It's not uncommon to *think* you aren't hungry—nothing sounds good, you could "take it or leave it" when it comes to food—but eventually consume a balanced meal without distress. I encourage meal planning to include foods you enjoy, family favorites, and occasional treats to look forward to. While it can be nice to never want to eat, silencing all joy from food is not the goal.

Constipation. GLP-1 medications work in many ways, but one is slowing digestion. This means that less frequent bowel movements are normal. If your stools are still easy-to-pass solid logs and feel complete, this will probably just be your new normal. If, however, you are bloated and uncomfortable and your stools are difficult to pass, you may need to add some tools. Gradually increasing high-fiber foods, drinking more fluids, and walking after meals are the first steps. Still not going? Ask your provider if they think an over-the-counter magnesium supplement, MiraLAX and/or Metamucil (psyllium husk) could help.

Diarrhea. Much less common but still a potential side effect, diarrhea can be difficult to manage. It's likely triggered by very high-fat or high-sugar foods and, for some, artificial sweeteners. Although there isn't much we can eat to stop diarrhea once it starts, it is important to stay well hydrated, so an electrolyte supplement fluid is recommended. Applesauce, bananas, broths, and simple carbohydrate foods, like saltine crackers, can help. Imodium might also help if your prescriber agrees it is safe for you. Adding fermented foods once you feel better, like kombucha, miso, sauerkraut, sourdough bread, tempeh, and yogurt, will support a healthy gut moving forward.

Fatigue. Feeling exhausted is not normal. Most people who are eating enough feel energetic on GLP-1 medications. If you're experiencing fatigue, needing extra naps, unable to make it through a usual day of activities, you are probably either dehydrated or severely undereating. I recommend adding easy-to-digest simple carbohydrates to your day—fruit snack bars, white rice or pasta, toast, juice, and electrolytes with your beverages.

Nausea and vomiting. In my experience, the primary causes of nausea while on a GLP-1 medication are high-fat foods, overly large meals, and skipping meals. Avoiding high-fat foods, even the "healthy ones," should help. Drinking ice-cold fluids, eating smaller, more frequent meals, and eating more slowly are also helpful tips. A little queasiness that is short-lived and manageable is normal. If your nausea prevents you from eating or drinking or is so severe that you are vomiting, reach out to your prescriber. Zofran, an antinausea prescription medication, may be an option. An over-the-counter B6 supplement can help too.

Reflux. Late-night meals and then lying down flat are the usual triggers for overnight reflux, although this can still occur during the day after larger, higher fat or spicy meals. If reflux is a problem for you, then consider avoiding alcohol, chocolate, citrus, spicy peppers, tobacco, and tomatoes and keeping meals smaller and lower in fat. Again, ask your provider if an over-the-counter acid-reducing medication is recommended for you.

Very low appetite. It's normal, especially when first starting your medication, to feel very full very quickly on very little food. While a few days of undereating here and there, especially immediately after shot day, is fine, it's important that you eat enough to have good energy and meet your basic nutrition needs. Eat low-fat foods to avoid feeling too full. Raw fruits and vegetables can also be avoided in the short term, as they can be too filling when appetite is low. Consider adding easily digestible simple carbs and electrolytes with your hydration. If you make it through breakfast and lunch but then are too full to eat dinner, look at your meal timing. Eat breakfast as early as possible, lunch at midday, and then try for a light dinner.

WHEN TO INCREASE YOUR DOSE

Knowing when to adjust your GLP-1 medication dosage is crucial for getting the most out of your treatment. Hopefully, you'll have a supportive and informed care team that can help guide you. It's important to recognize that the initial doses of the titration schedule are intended to be the "loading doses." Many patients will need to increase their dose month after month to the higher, more effective doses before they experience benefits.

First, evaluate how you feel. If side effects have become manageable after a few weeks but you're still not losing weight, it might be time to increase your dose. If you've hit a plateau, experience more food noise, or your weight isn't budging despite eating well and moving with intention, a higher dose could be helpful. Please know, however, that there is no reason to rush to increase your dose if you are having bothersome side effects, losing weight quickly, or struggling to eat enough to feel your best! Remember, we are not chasing the fastest weight loss possible; we want to lose weight safely while staying healthy.

KEEPING TRACK OF YOUR WEIGHT CHANGES

When you're on GLP-1 medications, tracking your weight can help you gauge how well the treatment is working. Most people start to see some weight loss within the first few weeks or months, while others may require dose increases to see the full benefit. Your goal should be about a 1 percent body weight loss (from your starting weight) per week across the course of your journey. Any faster and there's concern about muscle and bone loss, in addition to malnutrition.

TACKLING THE RETURN OF CRAVINGS

Many people notice that old cravings and food thoughts, that "food noise" we talked about, can come back after eight to twelve months of GLP-1 therapy. This is normal, unfortunately. *Despite this, people do maintain their weight loss!* If you find yourself battling these cravings again, there are nutrition strategies that can help. Eating a balanced diet and not skipping meals are key! Also, monitor your stress levels and sleep, as disruptions here can often trigger those pesky food thoughts. Make sure to have an open dialogue with your doctor too. They may want to adjust your dose or look at adding or trying other medications to help.

NAVIGATING MEDICATION SHORTAGES AND CONSIDERING COMPOUNDS

Increasing demand for GLP-1 medications and periodic supply shortages have left many patients with gaps in treatment and scrambling for alternatives. Navigating the complexities—unprecedented demand as health care providers increasingly recognize their effectiveness coupled with disruptions in the manufacturing and distribution processes due to global events and resource limitations—of these shortages raises important questions about access, safety, and potential substitute therapies, including compounded options.

In the face of shortages, some patients may consider compounded medications as an alternative to commercially available GLP-1 products. In the face of drug shortages, compounding pharmacies can legally create a similar formulation. However, these medications often lack the rigorous testing and standardization required for commercial products. Patients still need a prescription and should consult their health care providers before exploring compounded options. I cannot in good conscience recommend the purchase or use of "research peptides" bought online without a prescription.

The regulation of compounded medications varies by state and national guidelines, and patients should be aware of safety measures in place to protect them. In

COMPOUNDED MEDICATIONS

Compounded medications are custom-made prescriptions prepared by pharmacists to meet the unique needs of individual patients. Unlike mass-produced drugs, these medications are tailored to specific dosages, formulations, or ingredients that may not be commercially available. Compounding pharmacies have traditionally served patients with allergies to certain ingredients or those who need a medication in a different form, such as a liquid, cream, or flavored version. Patients typically access compounded medications through a prescription from their doctor, filling it at a licensed compounding pharmacy.

PRO TIP

There are two main types of compounding pharmacies: 503A and 503B.

A **503A compounding pharmacy** should only provide customized medications for individual patients based on a valid prescription from a licensed health care provider made to order on a per-patient basis.

A **503B compounding pharmacy** can operate as an "outsourcing facility," which allows them to produce large batches of compounded medications without specific patient prescriptions. Unlike 503A, the 503B facilities **are** regulated by the FDA and held to stricter standards to ensure the safety and quality of the medications produced at a larger scale.

the United States, the compounding of medications is overseen by state pharmacy boards and the FDA. Some manufacturers are actively pursuing lawsuits against compounding pharmacies, arguing that these pharmacies are infringing on their trademarks or misrepresenting their products. Such legal actions reflect the ongoing tension between the need for accessible treatment options during shortages and the necessity for pharmaceutical companies to protect their intellectual property and ensure the integrity of their products.

Patients should seek compounded medications from reputable pharmacies with robust oversight and certification. This can include verifying compliance with recognized compounding standards, such as those set forth by the Pharmacy Compounding Accreditation Board (PCAB). Additionally, patients should consider asking their health care providers about the pharmacy's reputation and reliability to mitigate any risks associated with compounded treatments. Open communication with health care providers is crucial during this time. Let your provider know when you cannot source your medicine and discuss potential alternatives.

The ongoing shortages of GLP-1 medications highlight broader systemic issues within the health care landscape, including the need for better supply chain management and contingency planning for high-demand medications. Advocacy for policies prioritizing equitable access to essential medications can help mitigate these shortages in the future, ensuring all patients can access the therapies they need.

COMPOUNDED GLP-1 SAFETY

Compounded GLP-1s are most often dispensed in multi-dose vials, which can potentially increase your safety risks. Here are some important tips to ensure your safety on compounded GLP-1s:

- These are usually delivered to your door by mail, so it is important that you ensure they arrive cold and are stored properly.

- Always use the recommended prescribed dose and schedule as ordered by your provider.

- Ensure that you understand the way the dosing is described on your prescription and compare that to the information on the vials and syringes provided. You may see different measurements such as "units," "ml," and/or "mg," which can be confusing and require you to do some math!

- Always reach out to your provider or pharmacy for clarification before administering a dose that may be incorrect.

- Because you will access the top of your vial more than once, it is important to use proper aseptic techniques and wipe the vial with an alcohol pad before inserting the needle.

- Be sure to discard open vials after the recommended time (usually twenty-eight days).

- Do not share your medication with others.

- Do report any adverse events, side effects, or concerns to both your provider and the pharmacy with which you sourced your medication.

CHAPTER 05

DEVELOPING YOUR NEW NUTRITION AND MOVEMENT PHILOSOPHY

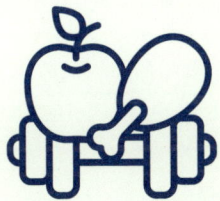

I know, I know, you want a scheme. You want a clear-cut, guaranteed plan. You want details and macros and calories and complicated hacks. Well, you think you want that. I know you think that losing weight is impossible without rules. And it probably was before GLP-1s. Remember, these medicines work by helping you navigate the real world with an appetite that is appropriately satisfied on reasonable amounts of food. That elusive calorie deficit required to shed pounds just happens (for most people) without a complicated plan.

Now, don't get it twisted, I'm not saying nutrition doesn't matter. It's just that we can now focus on the basics like quality, sustainability, enjoyability, and nutrient density without the exhausting work of forcing a deficit. It's honestly quite freeing!

STRUCTURED MINDFULNESS

As a registered dietitian (but also a human with a lifetime of experience struggling with my weight and food), I wish to present an evidence-based approach to health that diverges from conventional dieting paradigms. I've taken all the awesome knowledge I've learned from papers and textbooks and paired that with all the awesome lived experiences shared with me while working with others. While I can absolutely understand the comfort many of us find in a structured program, I notice, often, we tend to let go of our intuition along the way. So, in the spirit of avoiding black-and-white, all-or-nothing thinking, I'd like to coin a phrase that feels more nuanced.

Far too often I see plans that are either super strict or super intuitive—and I'm not a fan of either! I'm calling this new approach **structured mindfulness**, words that a dear client used to describe her takeaway after working with me. This method encourages a fundamental shift in perspective and behavior, fostering sustainable and holistic health improvements. It's both "touchy-feely" for the individual to apply and "scientifically aligned" to nutrition principles we know are healthful. It's structured in terms of meeting nutritional targets to ensure good health, but mindful in terms of honoring your hunger cues and eating all the foods you love!

TRANSITIONING FROM RESTRICTION TO ADEQUACY

The initial step in adopting structured mindfulness is transitioning from a mindset rooted in *restriction* to one oriented around *adequacy*. Traditional diets frequently emphasize exclusion—no carbs, low fats, no dairy, no grains, no gluten, no sugar, no meat, no fun, no joy—leading to poorly balanced intakes, confusion, misinformation, and limited adherence. Often the plans we take on slash calories so low we just feel, well, low on calories. Low-calorie plans are only sustainable for so long before our bodies fight back, get hungry, and overdo it. The negative psychological impact of "messing up" further discourages us from trying again. "Dieting" often follows a very unfair but predictable cycle of overeating and weight gain.

Instead, structured mindfulness requires you to ask yourself this question: "What does my body require to feel its best?" This approach is supported by research that shows that consuming nutrient-dense foods (foods high in fiber, vitamins, minerals, healthy fats, proteins, and complex carbohydrates) and attending to hunger signals (being satisfied) can lead to improved nutritional intake and meal satisfaction. Focusing on adequacy—and *feeling* adequately fed—promotes overall well-being by providing the necessary nutrients the body needs to function optimally (and improve our health).

"The best diet is the one you can stick to" is a quote you've probably heard. Not only does the way you eat meet your nutritional needs to help you feel your best and achieve your goals, but you can also continue to implement the plan while overcoming challenges and setbacks without feeling like you're moving a mountain to make *it* happen.

REJECTING THE ALL-OR-NOTHING MENTALITY: THE EFFICACY OF INCREMENTAL CHANGES

A significant barrier to lasting health and weight loss success is the all-or-nothing mentality pervasive in many diet plans. These protocols often advocate for strict compliance, creating unrealistic expectations and cycles of guilt upon deviation. Structured mindfulness, conversely, underscores the importance of *incremental adjustments*. Small, gradual changes—such as introducing an additional serving of vegetables to each meal or incorporating brief daily physical activity—can cumulatively yield substantive health benefits over time. Compounding small behavior improvements often leads to growing returns. It's a common misconception that big outcomes require big or extreme changes. Sure, losing 100 pounds (45.4 kg) sounds like it takes a massive effort from Day 1, when really you only lose 100 pounds (45.5 kg) after losing just 1 pound (454 g), 100 times. A lot of us have this bad habit of looking at big goals and deciding that because they're so big they're going to be hard, and because they're hard, we hesitate. But breaking down goals and the behaviors we want to change into small, manageable pieces supports durable habit formation through flexibility and self-compassion, which are crucial for long-term adherence and overall satisfaction.

Self-compassion is an often overlooked yet critical component in traditional weight loss narratives. Embracing self-compassion involves recognizing and accepting your imperfections without judgment, fostering a supportive and motivational environment within your mind. Weight stigma and shaming (from external or internal sources) do not motivate individuals to lose weight; instead, they are shown to increase stress, emotional eating, and an avoidance of physical activity. Research suggests that individuals who practice self-compassion are more likely to recover from setbacks and engage in healthier, more consistent behaviors. This is because self-compassion reduces the detrimental effects of shame and guilt, which can otherwise perpetuate a cycle of negative self-talk and unhealthy coping mechanisms. By treating yourself with kindness and understanding, you can better navigate the inevitable weight loss challenges, maintain a positive outlook, and sustain long-term health goals. TL;DR: small steps; be nice.

UTILIZING PAST EXPERIENCES TO INFORM DECISIONS

In a society heavily influenced by diet culture, rejecting its unhelpful principles is a necessary step toward genuine health improvement. Diet culture's emphasis on rapid results and unattainable body standards often result in short-term solutions, weight cycling, and disappointment. That's not to say you didn't learn a thing or two along the way. Tracking calories in an app may have increased your awareness and improved your intentionality. Your attempt at veganism for health may have improved your acceptance of vegetables or added new recipes to your repertoire. Your brief low-carb period probably helped you learn how to meet your protein needs with more than just meat. That personal trainer you hired may have written you a terrible meal plan, but he really did improve your squat form! *It's okay to look back on previous diets and find positives.*

Structured mindfulness encourages critical reflection on past dietary experiences to inform future practices. By incorporating insights from previous dietary attempts into a more mindful eating framework—recognizing overeating triggers and responding appropriately to hunger and satiety cues—you will be able to work toward sustainable weight management and healthier eating habits. For example, my time counting macros means I'm pretty good at making sure I'm getting enough protein without having to use an app—not that there's anything wrong with tracking (more on that later). This reflective practice enables a tailored approach to nutrition that integrates both your personal history and preferences for more effective and lasting outcomes.

REMINDER: ALL FOODS FIT

The concept that "all foods fit" within a balanced nutrition plan stems from the principle of dietary inclusivity, where no particular food is completely off-limits.

This approach is rooted in the understanding that labeling foods as "good" or "bad" can foster an unhealthy relationship with eating, leading to feelings of guilt and restriction. Biologically, incorporating a wide variety of foods ensures a more diverse intake of nutrients necessary for optimal health. Adding planned, occasional indulgences with sweets or savory snacks can mitigate feelings of deprivation; and it's this deprivation—not the food itself—that eventually results in overeating. Truly believing that all foods can be part of a healthy diet when consumed in appropriate portions promotes a more balanced and sustainable approach to nutrition and a more positive relationship with food.

THE CHALLENGE WITH MODERATION AND HOW GLP-1s MAKE THIS POSSIBLE

While the mantra "everything in moderation" or "all foods fit" (in appropriate portions) is widely accepted in our vernacular, practicing that moderation can be extremely challenging for many individuals, particularly those with dysregulated appetite control and metabolic health. Before starting my GLP-1 journey, I truly thought the "intuitive eating" folks were full of shit! Turns out, they just don't have the same biological dysfunctions that I do! For some of us, the interplay of genetic, biological, metabolic, psychological, environmental, and situational factors may make it difficult to regulate portion sizes and frequency of consumption of certain foods (*or all foods, even*). This is where glucagon-like peptide-1 (GLP-1) receptor agonists come into play—significantly aiding in weight reduction partly by making it easier to adhere to the practice of moderation. By modulating the body's natural hunger signals, these medications help individuals better control their food intake without the constant struggle against hunger, facilitating a more manageable and sustainable approach to weight management. Instead of feeling as though you have to eat the entire pack of Oreos, two are plenty satisfying!

TO TRACK OR NOT TO TRACK: BALANCING AWARENESS WITH OBSESSION

The debate over whether to track food intake is contentious among nutrition professionals and the public at large, as it presents both potential benefits and drawbacks. Tracking can provide valuable data, making you more aware of eating patterns and helping you make informed choices—a practice supported by research consistently finding that nutrition self-monitoring is associated with more significant weight loss. Tools like calorie-counting apps and food journals can help identify nutritional opportunities and guide portion control decisions and practice.

However, for some of us, meticulous tracking can shift into an unhealthy obsession, contributing to anxiety and disordered eating behaviors. The key is to approach tracking with flexibility, using it as a tool for awareness rather than as a rigid rulebook. I always say there is no A+ or F- grade for tracking, and unless you have a dietitian reviewing your logs, most of us just track for ourselves; doing it perfectly or doing it imperfectly doesn't matter. The true benefit of tracking comes from the consistency of tracking as a habit, holding yourself accountable to your goals. If you're the type that tracks for one meal and then not again for days, that's probably not helpful. If you're only tracking your healthiest days, also, who cares. If you're gonna track, track. Track. It. All. You are not a good or bad person based on the foods you eat or the consistency with which you track your meals—it's just data. However, if you're prone to obsessive or restrictive food behaviors, tracking is probably only going to add stress and frustration to your life. Taking a balanced and nonjudgmental approach to self-monitoring ensures that tracking supports, rather than undermines, overall mental and physical well-being.

THE IMPORTANCE OF NUTRIENT DENSITY ON GLP-1 MEDICATIONS

Focusing on nutrient density (instead of restriction) is key when utilizing GLP-1 medications to treat obesity. When you're just unable to eat a lot, eating nutritiously matters more. *Nutrient-dense foods are foods that provide high levels of vitamins, minerals, and other beneficial compounds relative to their calorie content.* Prioritizing foods such as lean proteins, fruits, vegetables, and whole grains helps ensure that your diet supports overall health despite the reduced calorie intakes induced by GLP-1 medications.

CREATING SYSTEMS TO SUPPORT CHANGE

To maximize the benefits of GLP-1 medications, consider implementing supportive systems. Meal planning can streamline grocery shopping, ensure nutritional balance, and reduce the temptation to make unhealthy food choices. Planning ahead allows you to create a nutrient-dense menu tailored to your dietary needs and

ADDITIONAL SUPPORT SYSTEMS YOU CAN TRY

- Accountability buddies
- App-based behavior trackers
- Consistent exercise schedule
- Hiring a personal trainer
- Local Community Supported Agriculture (CSA) vegetable memberships
- Meal delivery programs
- Meditation
- Online communities
- Reflective journaling
- Regular visits with a registered dietitian
- Support groups
- Structured morning and bedtime routines

preferences. People who regularly plan their meals in advance are more likely to consume a wider variety of foods, meet dietary guidelines, and maintain a healthy weight. Incorporating meal planning into your routine fosters consistency and reduces the mental burden associated with daily food decisions.

EATING ENOUGH ON PURPOSE PREVENTS OVEREATING BY ACCIDENT

One critical aspect of managing appetite with GLP-1 medications is ensuring you consume adequate nourishment intentionally. Skipping meals or undereating can lead to unintended overeating, the return of food noise, and frustration undermining your weight management efforts. Regular, balanced meals help maintain steady blood sugar levels and prevent unmanageable hunger. By deliberately planning and consuming nutrient-rich meals, you can avoid restrictive and reactive eating behaviors and sustain a stable, manageable relationship with food.

SEEKING SATIETY VS. AVOIDING HUNGER

There's a significant difference between seeking satiety and merely avoiding hunger. Seeking satiety involves choosing foods that sustain fullness and provide lasting energy. Foods high in protein, fiber, and healthy fats most effectively prolong satiety and energy. But satisfaction is about more than just physical fullness—you *deserve* to enjoy the food too! Foods that are flavorful, colorful, or cultural improve the perception of satiety! In contrast, merely avoiding hunger, ignoring it, or seeking to never feel it might lead to selecting less nutritious meal options.

DIMINISHING RETURNS ON "DIET PERFECTION"

Striving for a perfect diet can lead to frustration and burnout, ultimately acting as a barrier to success rather than as a benefit or motivator. Overly rigid dietary restrictions are often unsustainable and can lead to cyclical patterns of restriction and binge eating. Understanding that diminishing returns exist on dietary perfection allows more flexibility and sustainability in eating habits. The perfect diet does not ensure more weight loss or better health. There really is such a thing as *good enough*. I truly believe that good nutrition lives on a continuum where there is always room for improvement and decline. (And we will ebb and flow along the continuum depending on our circumstances!) Your focus should be on overall dietary patterns and consistently eating nutrient-dense foods rather than adhering to an unattainable ideal. Macro habits, our overarching patterns of behavior, play a much more significant role in health outcomes than obsessing over micro details. Establishing foundational habits such as regular physical activity, consistent meal planning, and self-compassion has been shown to have a more substantial impact on long-term health than focusing on the minute dietary details.

THE POWER OF MOVEMENT

In today's health landscape, we often hear about the "importance of diet and exercise," mostly as a method for *weight loss*. But movement is fundamental to human biology and health.

Historically, our ancestors relied on physical activity for survival, whether hunting for food or escaping danger. In our modern society, though, the necessity of movement has diminished, leading to negative health outcomes resulting from sedentary lifestyles. It is vital to understand, though, that the benefits of exercise extend far beyond weight loss. By shifting the focus away from weight loss, you can explore movement as a means of self-care, personal empowerment, and getting strong.

PRO TIP

To see a true picture of your body composition (muscle mass, fat distribution, and bone density), a DEXA scan (dual-energy X-ray absorptiometry) is the gold standard. You can usually find one in a commercial gym or wellness center in your area for about $150 USD. I recommend getting a scan at three- to six-month intervals to ensure you are losing body fat (not muscle) along this journey!

In addition to boosting metabolism, regular physical activity enhances insulin sensitivity, helping regulate blood sugar levels and reducing the risk of type 2 diabetes. Moreover, engaging in regular movement can help reduce chronic inflammation, which is linked to numerous diseases including cardiovascular disease and certain cancers. Regular movement promotes flexibility, which is critical for maintaining mobility as we age. Balance exercises can also help prevent falls, enhancing confidence in daily activities. Additionally, maintaining muscle strength and mobility is vital for independence, allowing individuals to navigate their environments, engage socially, and retain autonomy.

The benefits of movement extend beyond the physiological and include psychological well-being too—exercise can improve mental health. Regular physical activity stimulates the release of endorphins, those "feel-good hormones." Studies have shown a positive correlation between regular exercise and reduced levels of anxiety and depression. Additionally, exercise has been shown to foster neurogenesis—the creation of new brain cells—and improve cognitive functions, like attention, memory, and executive functioning skills. Regular physical activity also decreases the body's stress hormones, such as cortisol, while stimulating the production of neurotransmitters that promote relaxation and improve mood. Individuals who prioritize mobility often report higher levels of satisfaction and happiness in their daily lives.

MUSCLE IS MEDICINE

Intentional movement helps maintain and improve muscle mass, which is crucial as we age. Muscle is metabolically active tissue that plays a significant role in our overall health and metabolism. As we increase strength training and physical activity, we build muscle mass, which enhances our resting metabolic rate (RMR). A higher resting metabolic rate means our body burns more calories at rest, making it easier to maintain a healthy body composition. Studies show that even small increases in muscle mass, and preventing its loss as we age, can lead to improved length and quality of life.

BODY COMPOSITION

When discussing movement and muscle, body composition also plays a prominent role in overall health outcomes. Understanding body composition—the ratio of fat to lean mass—provides insights into metabolic health. Higher lean muscle mass is directly linked to a reduced risk of chronic diseases. Research has consistently demonstrated that increases in muscle mass can improve overall health markers, including lower blood pressure, better cholesterol profiles, and improved glucose metabolism. It's also important to consider body fat distribution, not only the total amount of body fat but also where that fat is stored on your body. Visceral fat, stored around the organs, is particularly harmful and has been associated with various health issues such as heart disease and diabetes. Fat around the hips and thighs? Not as worrisome!

In my opinion, body composition is more important for long-term health than the number on the scale, and most people are "undermuscled." Although I think the risk of muscle loss while on a GLP-1 is somewhat overhyped in the mainstream

HEALTHY BODY FAT PERCENTAGE GOALS

Men

- Ages 20 to 39: 8 to 19 percent
- Ages 40 to 59: 11 to 21 percent
- Ages 60 to 79: 13 to 24 percent

Women

- Ages 20 to 39: 21 to 32 percent
- Ages 40 to 59: 23 to 33 percent
- Ages 60 to 79: 24 to 35 percent

PRO TIP

The goal isn't to eliminate **all** body fat. Yes, excess body fat can contribute to poor health, but an adequate amount of body fat is essential for several important bodily functions, such as:

- Biological function: Maintaining healthy brain function, mood regulation, and cognitive performance

- Energy storage: Reserves that come in handy in times of fasting, famine, illness, and injury

- Fat-soluble nutrient absorption: Of vitamins A, D, E, and K and storage to prevent deficiencies

- Hormone production: Particularly critical in women to maintain fertility

- Physical protection: Of organs and bones from trauma or injury

- Temperature regulation: An insulating layer vital for maintaining a stable internal environment, especially in colder conditions

media, it is real. Losing weight too quickly, regardless of the method, without strength training, is not a good idea.

Now, strength training is a broad term that can include a wide variety of exercise modalities. Most people immediately think of weight lifting, but resistance training can include functional fitness, hiking, Pilates, resistance bands, swimming, yoga, and more. The key is to push your physical abilities beyond your current level, moving in a way that is challenging, and then continuing to progress those movements to make them more challenging as you get stronger. I believe most women do not lift heavy enough. But, just like any other healthy habit, these are skills we have to practice. I highly recommend hiring a personal trainer (if this is accessible to you). Building confidence in the gym is also a skill, and you don't have to do it alone! Finding something you enjoy and making it a habit is more important than doing whatever is "best." And remember, working out for 10 minutes a day, every day, is far more beneficial than working out for 2 hours once a week. Start small and build on your progress with time and consistency!

IMPROVING FITNESS ON GLP-1s

You may be thinking that while on a GLP-1 medication you just won't be able to eat enough to support your fitness routine. Aside from just feeling better and increasing motivation to do the thing, if we think about the science and benefits behind how these medications work, we find that GLP-1s actually can support us in becoming the athletes we want to be. Here, I will take you through all the ways that taking a GLP-1 can actually improve your fitness.

- Maintaining stable blood sugar levels is critical for optimal athletic performance. Fluctuations in blood sugar can lead to energy crashes, reduced endurance, and impaired recovery. By enhancing insulin sensitivity and stabilizing blood sugar levels, GLP-1s can provide a more consistent energy supply during workouts, potentially improving endurance and overall performance.

- For athletes and fitness enthusiasts, achieving a healthy body weight can enhance relative strength, reduce the risk of injuries, and improve endurance. Lower body fat percentages are often associated with increased agility and speed, crucial for athletic performance.

- Cardiovascular health is also fundamental for sustaining prolonged physical activity and enhancing performance. GLP-1s have been shown to offer protective cardiovascular benefits, including reducing blood pressure and improving lipid profiles. Better cardiovascular health translates to improved aerobic capacity, allowing athletes to train harder, perform stronger, and recover faster.

- Inflammation is a natural response to intense physical activity, but chronic or excessive inflammation can hinder performance and recovery. There is evidence suggesting GLP-1s have anti-inflammatory properties, which may help reduce muscle soreness and accelerate recovery times. Faster recovery allows for more frequent and intense training sessions, ultimately leading to greater performance gains.

- Lastly, GLP-1s may improve the uptake of glucose by muscle cells, providing an immediate source of energy during physical exertion. This enhanced glucose uptake can support sustained high-intensity performance and delay the onset of fatigue. Efficient glucose use during exercise is critical for activities that require bursts of power, such as sprinting or weightlifting.

So, the takeaway here: Let's *goooo!*

PREVENTING INJURY FOR LONG-TERM SUCCESS

I encourage you to approach this fitness journey with a realistic mindset that ensures long-term success and avoids the pitfalls that can lead to injuries. Understanding the importance of starting slow and implementing injury-prevention techniques can improve your ability to maintain longevity and consistency in your exercise routine. One of the most common mistakes beginners make is diving into a new workout regimen too intensely, which can put undue stress on the body. While enthusiasm is a good thing, it's important to recognize that our body needs time to adapt to new physical demands. Remember:

- Progress is personal: Everyone's fitness journey is unique. Celebrate your progress, no matter how small, and avoid comparing yourself to others.
- Be patient: Change doesn't happen overnight. Trust the process and understand that gradual, consistent effort will lead to lasting results.
- Stay educated: Continuously learning about new workout techniques, nutrition, and injury-prevention strategies empowers you to make informed decisions.

LET'S TALK ABOUT WALKING

Walking offers substantial health benefits that contribute to an improved quality of life. Engaging in consistent walking routines can lead to better cardiovascular health, mood enhancement, and cognitive function. Walking at a moderate pace can effectively lower blood pressure, improve cholesterol levels, and support overall heart health. In addition to physical benefits, walking significantly affects mental well-being. It has been linked to reductions in depression and anxiety symptoms while also promoting an increase in overall happiness. The rhythmic and repetitive nature of walking produces a calming effect, making it an excellent activity for stress relief.

Setting step goals, such as the popular target of 10,000 steps per day, provides a tangible benchmark for physical activity. While the origin of the 10,000 steps goal

A COMPREHENSIVE APPROACH TO FITNESS

A comprehensive approach to fitness might include a little something from each category on a regular cadence:

- Everyday activities that interrupt sedentary time: play, housekeeping, gardening, dog walking, dancing

- High-intensity movement: spin class, running, high-intensity interval training (HIIT)

- Low-intensity weight-bearing movement: walking, swimming, hiking

- Mobility and flexibility: stretching, foam rolling

- Strength training: yoga, weight lifting, resistance bands, Pilates, body weight exercises

can be traced back to a Japanese marketing campaign (Fun fact: 10k in Japanese looks like a person walking!) rather than scientific evidence, it has become a globally accepted standard. Recent research, however, suggests that even smaller step targets, like 7,000 to 8,000 steps per day, can offer substantial health benefits, particularly for older adults. The rise of wearable technology has revolutionized step tracking, making it easier than ever to monitor daily activity levels. Devices such as fitness trackers, pedometers, and smartphones equipped with step-counting features provide real-time feedback and motivation. This immediate data fosters a sense of accomplishment and encourages consistent movement, helping people stay on track with their fitness goals.

Critics of the emphasis on step counts, however, argue that focusing solely on the number of steps can be overly simplistic. Health benefits are also influenced by factors such as the speed, resistance, and intensity of the steps. Solely emphasizing step counts may lead some to overlook other important components of a well-rounded fitness regimen, such as lifting weights. It's crucial to adopt a comprehensive approach that considers various aspects of physical health. As we age, it's better to do a little bit of everything than to specialize in any specific modality!

While going for a long walk in the morning and calling it a day sounds appealing, it is actually more important to intentionally reduce sedentary time throughout the day. Prolonged sitting has been linked to heightened risks of chronic diseases and increased mortality rates, regardless of overall physical activity levels. Integrating short walks or standing breaks into daily routines can mitigate some of these risks by breaking up long periods of inactivity.

THE CONFLICT BETWEEN PERFORMANCE AND WEIGHT LOSS

In the pursuit of a healthier lifestyle, a lot of us tend to set a variety of goals beyond the scale. Among the most common are improving fitness and enhancing performance, all while hoping to lose weight. Understanding how these goals intersect—and how the choices we make to achieve them can affect our progress—helps us maintain a balanced and healthy approach to fitness.

One of the primary areas where fitness goals can clash with weight loss objectives is in the realm of performance. Whether you are a runner, a weightlifter, or engage in any athletic activities with measurable outcomes, your body requires a certain amount of fuel to perform at its best. This fuel, primarily derived from the calories and nutrients you consume, is essential not only for energy but also for recovery and injury prevention. To perform at high levels, athletes need adequate caloric intake. This includes plenty of carbohydrates for energy, protein for muscle repair and growth, and fats for health and recovery. When the focus shifts to weight loss, caloric intake is often reduced, sometimes so significantly that performance suffers.

As body weight decreases, it's not uncommon to see a drop in absolute strength—the amount of weight one can lift. This happens because losing weight often means losing some muscle mass along with fat. And, well, *mass moves mass*. Bigger folks have physics on their side! For those who prioritize performance, this can be particularly disheartening, as lifting heavier weights or achieving personal records may become more challenging. However, it's important to remember the concept of *relative strength*, which is the amount of weight lifted relative to body weight. While absolute strength (how much you can lift regardless of body weight) may decrease as you lose weight, relative strength can improve. This means that although you might be lifting lighter absolute weights, the weight you are lifting compared to your body weight can be higher, potentially improving your efficiency and performance in movements that require you to move your body weight, such as pull-ups or jumping.

Balancing performance and fitness goals with weight loss can be challenging, but it is certainly achievable with a mindful and informed approach. By making intentional choices about nutrition, training, and recovery, you can work toward a healthier, stronger body without sacrificing (too much) performance. Remember, the journey to fitness and health is a marathon, not a sprint, and finding the right balance supports long-term success and well-being.

CHAPTER 06

EATING WELL AND STAYING HYDRATED

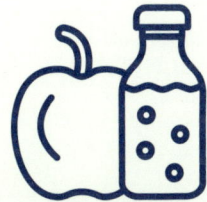

Before we dive into the details of how to structure your nutrition and food choices, understand that there really isn't a "special diet" just because you are taking a GLP-1 medication. If you've made it this far in this book and are disappointed to learn that I'm not hiding a special secret in this chapter, I apologize. The thing is, the GLP-1s just make it easier to stick to the usual recommendations for a balanced and nutritious eating pattern. Instead of stressing over calories, ingredients, or some novel nutrition approach, we can find some structure to our nutrition that supports good health—and sustainable weight loss—without falling prey to extremism or overrestriction.

In the quest for weight management and improved overall health, many people focus on individual food choices, becoming preoccupied with whether a certain item is "healthy" or "unhealthy." However, most dietitians agree that the patterns and overall context of the meals we consume are far more important than the individual foods themselves.

BALANCE MATTERS MORE THAN INDIVIDUAL FOODS

A balanced meal pattern includes adequate portions of macronutrients—carbohydrates, proteins, and fats—along with essential vitamins and minerals. Instead of fixating on individual foods, adopting a holistic view that encourages a variety of choices across all food groups leads to better health outcomes. Research consistently shows the benefits of balanced meal patterns rich in fruits, healthy fats, lean proteins, vegetables, and whole grains, resulting in better weight management and lower incidence of chronic diseases. Following a diverse diet allows not only for nutrient adequacy but also enjoyment!

SATISFACTION AND SUSTAINABILITY

Satisfaction from meals goes beyond feeling full; it encompasses both physical and emotional aspects. When meals are balanced, they provide the body with all the necessary nutrients it needs. But emotional satisfaction is equally important. Eating is often a social and cultural experience, and when individuals restrict themselves excessively or focus on certain foods as "bad," feelings of deprivation can result. We see often that very restrictive eating plans can backfire, triggering binge eating or extreme cravings, ultimately derailing weight management efforts. *The pursuit of balance over perfection builds consistency.* When we obsess over "good" versus "bad" foods, we create cognitive dissonance that can lead to guilt and shame associated with eating. A person fixated on strict caloric limits may choose low-calorie options but miss out on important nutrients, leaving them unsatisfied and more prone to cravings. Someone who emphasizes balanced meal patterns—prioritizing whole nutrient-dense foods—can better navigate social situations and stressful days without falling into the trap of deprivation. Ultimately, long-term health is not about tracking every calorie or making rigid distinctions between good and bad foods; it's about creating a positive relationship with food that prioritizes balance, satisfaction, and sustainability.

USING THE PLATE METHOD

The plate method is a simple and easy-to-visualize approach to nutrition and weight management that dates back to the early 1990s when it was first introduced by the American Diabetes Association (ADA) and later adopted by the US Department of

Agriculture (USDA) to replace the food pyramid. It was designed to help us control portion sizes and achieve a balanced diet without the need for complex calorie or carbohydrate counting. The method involves dividing a 9-inch (23 cm) plate into sections: half for nonstarchy vegetables, a quarter for lean protein, and a quarter for grains or starchy foods. It's simple—on purpose!

Your GLP-1 Plate

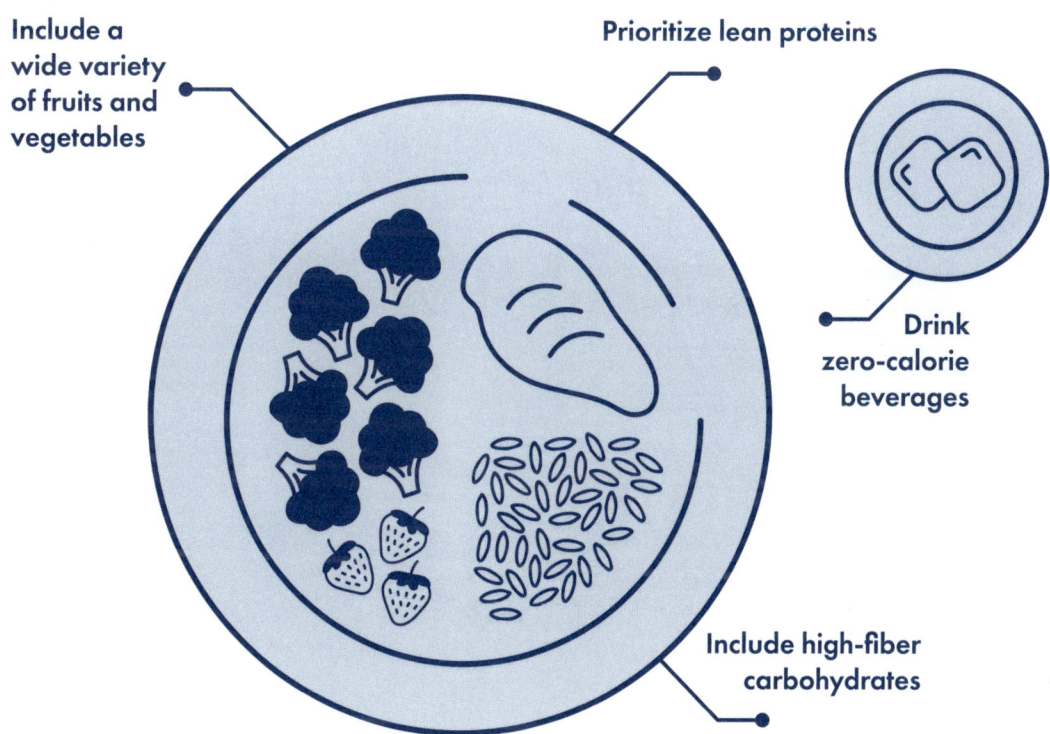

Include a wide variety of fruits and vegetables

Prioritize lean proteins

Drink zero-calorie beverages

Include high-fiber carbohydrates

Note: Portion sizes can be approximate and may vary day to day depending on your appetite or activities. Allow your GLP-1 medication, energy levels, and digestion to help guide your needs.

The benefits of the plate method include its ease of use, ability to encourage the consumption of various nutrients, and its adaptability to different cuisines and dietary needs. However, one drawback is that it does not provide precise control over calorie intake for people looking for an exacting approach. This simple, practical, and effective tool for promoting healthy eating habits and portion control is an excellent foundation for meal planning and food choices. When you no longer need to micromanage your nutrition to lose weight thanks to the appetite control provided by the medications, your job is simply to create a plate of food that is nourishing and balanced.

BALANCED MEAL FOR WEIGHT LOSS

- 4 to 6 ounces (115 to 170 g by weight) lean protein (provides roughly 20 to 30 grams of protein per serving)
- ½ cup (weight varies) complex carbohydrate food (such as whole grains, potatoes, pasta, or corn)
- 1 to 2 cups (weight varies) fruit and/or vegetables
- Flavor enhancers for fun (keeping added fats low, less than 1-ounce, or 28 g, servings for weight loss and GLP-1 tolerance)

BALANCED MEAL FOR MAINTENANCE

- 6 to 8 ounces (170 to 225 g by weight) lean protein (provides roughly 30 to 40 grams of protein per serving)
- 1 cup (weight varies) complex carbohydrate food
- 1 to 2 cups (weight varies) fruit and/or vegetables
- Flavor enhancers for fun (with a little more allowance for healthy fats as tolerated)

Unclear what foods fit into each category? Don't worry! We have lists and a sample meal plan for you in chapter 8!

LET'S TALK ABOUT CALORIES

It's not unusual for people to find themselves hyperfocused on calories over all else, especially while trying to lose weight. It's true, calories matter. It's also true that you have to be in a calorie deficit to lose weight. *This doesn't mean you have to count them.*

While a calorie is a measure of energy, the nutritional quality of foods contributing those calories varies greatly. For instance, 200 calories from a sugary soda provide quick energy but lack essential nutrients and can lead to blood sugar spikes, contributing to weight gain and very little satiety. Conversely, 200 calories from a nutrient-dense food, like almonds, offer protein, healthy fats, fiber, vitamins, and minerals, which promote satiety and provide sustained energy while supporting overall health.

Moreover, the body's metabolism processes macronutrients differently; proteins and fiber require more energy to digest and metabolize than refined carbohydrates. Therefore, focusing on the *quality and balance* of the foods you consume, rather than just caloric content, is necessary for maintaining long-term health, weight management, and well-being.

Determining your personal calorie needs involves several steps and considers various factors such as age, sex, weight, height, and physical activity level. I could tell you how to do this, but there are many great online calculators these days, so it would be a waste of space. And since we aren't going to track them, what's the point?

ACHIEVING A CALORIE DEFICIT

Achieving a calorie deficit, which is, unfortunately, essential for weight loss, can be accomplished through various methods, each with its unique pros and cons that depend on our individual preferences and skills.

> *Adopting a low-carb or ketogenic diet* can help some individuals lose weight but can feel restrictive and difficult to maintain long-term.

> *Calorie tracking* is popular, using a variety of apps or online food journals. The best use of these tools is for accuracy and consistency; you can then adjust based on weight trends.

Dietary modification, a common approach, reduces portion sizes or promotes choosing lower calorie foods, which directly reduces caloric intake. (This most aligns with our strategy here.)

Intermittent fasting is another strategy gaining popularity that simply cuts out entire meal periods, reducing calorie intake. *(I do not recommend this approach!)*

Regardless of the method you use, the most critical factor for success is adherence and consistency. Sustainable weight loss comes from finding a strategy that fits your lifestyle and preferences so you stick with it over time. My goal is to help it feel less difficult and emphasize that *your* chosen method should not feel overly restrictive or punishing, as this can lead to burnout and failure. Instead, small, manageable changes that gradually become part of a routine are more likely to result in lasting weight loss.

UNDERSTANDING MACRONUTRIENTS

In the realm of nutrition science, macronutrients hold center stage as the foundational pillars of our diet. Macronutrients include proteins, carbohydrates, and fats. Each macronutrient plays a vital role in maintaining our health, providing energy, and facilitating the myriad functions our body performs daily. It's important, though, to recognize that no one macronutrient is consumed in isolation; in reality, meals (and foods!) are usually a mix of carbohydrates, proteins, and fats. With that in mind, let's look at each of these essential nutrients to understand their core benefits and roles, including their caloric values and special considerations while on a GLP-1 medication.

PROTEIN

Proteins are the body's building blocks, vital for growth and repair. They play a critical role in the structure, function, and regulation of tissues and organs and are integral in forming enzymes, hormones, and antibodies, making them essential for immune function, muscle growth, and tissue repair. Proteins are composed of amino acids, some of which are essential, *meaning we must obtain them through our diet.* Each gram of protein provides approximately 4 calories. Foods such as dairy, poultry, seafood, legumes, meats, and nuts are rich in protein.

How Much Protein Do You Need on a GLP-1?

Determining the right amount of protein to consume is important and varies based on several factors, including age, sex, physical activity level, and overall health. The USDA's recommended dietary allowance (RDA) for protein generally stands at 0.8 grams of protein per kilogram of body weight for the average adult. This, however, has been greatly debated as much too low for most people.

GLP-1s get a bad rap for increasing the risk for muscle loss, and while this is a risk with any method of weight loss, it is still important to preserve as much muscle as possible. A high-protein diet coupled with regular resistance training does the trick.

For those individuals looking to achieve or maintain weight loss (and those who engage in regular physical activity), the requirement is much more—between 1.2 and 2.0 grams of protein per kilogram of body weight to support muscle repair and growth and keep you fuller longer! Of course, that 2.0g/kg may be unreachable in reality at our higher starting weights, especially if your appetite is suppressed. But you may be able to slowly creep closer to the high end of the range the closer you get to your goal.

The exact method used to ensure you "eat enough protein" doesn't really matter. Aiming for at least one-quarter of your plate filled with lean protein is likely enough. Some may prefer to track these macronutrients to ensure adequate intake and understand exactly where their protein comes from. While a few weeks of this can certainly be enlightening, this exactness isn't necessary. If you're intentional about including lean-protein foods at every meal and snack in large enough servings to meet your needs, you're likely "close enough." I recommend finding a ballpark range of protein goals, for example, 163 grams a day from the weight loss phase, and then divide that by the number of meals and snacks you plan to eat in a day.

163 g / 4 (3 meals + 1 snack) = 40.75 g of protein per meal—
the equivalent of approximately 5 ounces (140 g by weight) of chicken breast

DOING YOUR OWN PROTEIN MATH

Weight in pounds divided by 2.2 = weight in kilograms
Multiply your weight in kilograms by 0.8, 1.2, or 2.0 to get grams of protein
Example: 300 pounds / 2.2 = 136.36 kg

RDA: 136 × 0.8 = 109 g protein on very low hunger days (minimum)
Weight Loss Phase: 136 × 1.2 = 163 g protein
Maintenance Phase: If at a "goal weight," for example, 160 pounds, or 72.7 kg
72.7 × 2.0 = 145 g protein

Vegan and Vegetarian Proteins

You can absolutely achieve a healthy, high-protein, muscle-preserving diet while on a GLP-1 and being vegan or vegetarian. Vegan diets exclude all animal products, including dairy and eggs, whereas vegetarians may include these. A whole food plant based–leaning diet has shown incredible health benefits. There are ample sources of protein available for those following a vegan or vegetarian diet, although mindful planning ensures an adequate intake of all essential amino acids.

Vegan protein sources are diverse and include legumes such as black beans, chickpeas, kidney beans, and lentils. Nuts and seeds, including almonds, chia seeds, flaxseed, hemp seeds, and walnuts, offer protein and healthy fats. Grains, notably barley, farro, and quinoa, not only provide protein but also various essential nutrients. Soy products, such as tofu, tempeh, and edamame, are versatile, protein-rich options that can be incorporated into numerous dishes. See chapter 8 for more on lean protein options.

Vegetarians, on the other hand, can also incorporate dairy products rich in protein, like cheese, milk, and yogurt. For those who are lactose intolerant or prefer nondairy options, many fortified alternatives provide similar nutritional benefits. Soy and pea milk, offering 6 to 8 grams of protein per cup (235 ml), like cow's milk, are the highest protein nondairy milk options. Almond milk, coconut milk, and oat milk are not great sources of protein. Concerns about soy products and soy's effects on hormone levels due to phytoestrogens (plant compounds that mimic estrogen) have been largely debunked; moderate consumption of soy is safe for most people and can be part of a balanced diet and offer additional health benefits such as lowering cholesterol and preventing cancer.

Fish and Seafood

Fish and seafood are exceptional sources of complete protein, omega-3 fatty acids, and other essential nutrients. Consuming a variety of fish in your diet—at least twice per week is recommended—can provide significant health benefits, including support for heart function and anti-inflammatory effects. For instance, a 4-ounce (115 g by weight) serving of salmon provides approximately 31 grams of protein, making it a nutrient powerhouse. Tuna, another excellent option, offers about 32 grams of protein per 4-ounce (115 g by weight) serving. Recent improvements in aquaculture practices have produced farmed fish with nutritional profiles similar to their wild counterparts. There isn't much additional nutritional benefit to purchasing the more expensive options; any seafood is better than none! If sustainability is a concern, look for one of the sustainable seafood certifications: Best Aquaculture Practices (BAP) for farmed fish or Marine Stewardship Council (MSC) for wild-caught fish.

Protein Supplements

For those on GLP-1 medications with limited capacity to eat a lot of food, meeting daily protein requirements through food intake alone can be challenging. Protein supplements are a convenient and effective solution to ensuring adequate intake.
Various types of protein supplements cater to different needs.

- Casein protein, a dairy-based option, digests more slowly than whey, providing a steady release of amino acids and making it suitable for consumption before bed to support overnight recovery.

- Hemp protein, though slightly lower in overall protein content, contains all essential amino acids and is rich in omega-3 fatty acids.

- Pea protein, derived from yellow peas, is a plant-based, hypoallergenic protein source containing all essential amino acids, though it is slightly lower in certain branched-chain amino acids (BCAAs) essential for muscle repair and growth.

- Soy protein, comparable in quality to animal proteins, is another plant-based complete protein option.

- Whey protein, another dairy-based protein, is quickly absorbed and, as a complete protein, is high in BCAAs essential for muscle repair and growth.

When selecting a protein supplement, consider the source and personal dietary preferences; it's hard to say which protein is "better" than any other, just that they all offer benefits. It is also important to remember that protein supplements are not intended to replace solid foods or entire meals. Shakes and smoothies are best used as true supplemental additions to the day's meals to meet high protein targets when appetite is low. In fact, a common pitfall for those taking GLP-1s is overreliance on protein supplements and lack of variety in protein foods.

CARBOHYDRATES

You should not be restricting carbohydrates to unsustainable levels. You may need to be more mindful of them and practice smart portion control, but avoiding them you will not. I get it—as a person living in a larger body and likely struggling with insulin resistance, restricting carbohydrates may have been the only method of weight loss that ever "worked." But if going "low carb" really worked, would you be here—reading this book, considering or taking a GLP-1 medication? What if I told you that you could now eat carbohydrates, enjoy them, reap all the benefits, and still lose weight?

Carbohydrates, found in whole grains, rice, potatoes, pasta, and oats, are important for fueling daily activities. When consumed, carbohydrates break down into glucose, which is then used by the body's cells to produce energy. Each gram of carbohydrate provides about 4 calories. The most important reason to consume carbohydrates may be fiber, which promotes digestive health by aiding bowel movements and enhancing gut microbiota that enhance digestion, support vitamin absorption, and provide important signals to the immune system.

Simple vs. Complex Carbs

Carbohydrates can be broadly classified into two categories: simple and complex. Simple carbohydrates, or simple sugars, consist of one or two sugar molecules and are quickly absorbed by the body. Examples include fructose, glucose, and sucrose found in candies, fruits, and processed foods. They provide rapid energy but can lead to spikes and crashes in blood sugar levels. Complex carbohydrates consist of long chains of sugar molecules, taking longer to digest and offering sustained energy. They are found in foods like legumes, vegetables, and whole grains. Complex carbs also contain fiber, which aids digestion and contributes to feelings of fullness. Complex carbohydrates will support health and weight loss more than simple carbs. See chapter 8 for more complex carb options.

However, easily digested simple carbohydrates can be crucial during the acclimation phases of GLP-1 dosing. For instance, when experiencing nausea or gastrointestinal distress, bland, easily digested carbs, like crackers, toast, or white rice, can be soothing and less likely to irritate a sensitive stomach. For individuals with hypoglycemia (low blood sugar), consuming simple carbs can raise blood sugar levels quickly to a safe range. Foods like candy, fruit juice, or glucose tablets are commonly recommended in these instances for their rapid absorption and immediate energy boost, helping alleviate symptoms of confusion, dizziness, or shakiness.

PRO TIP

Carbohydrates are just as important for building muscle as protein. If proteins are the building blocks on the construction site that is your physique, carbohydrates are the bulldozers and dump trucks that carry those blocks where they need to go to be put to use.

High-Sugar Foods

Sugars are simple carbohydrates that provide quick energy. While naturally occurring sugars in dairy, fruits, and vegetables are part of a balanced diet, the added sugars found in processed foods can be detrimental, and we should limit them. When we consume high-sugar foods, our body experiences a rapid spike in blood glucose levels, triggering the pancreas to release insulin, a hormone necessary for glucose uptake in cells for energy production; for those *without* the chronic diseases of obesity or diabetes or with underlying insulin resistance, this metabolic process works well. However, consistent consumption of high-sugar foods can exacerbate underlying dysfunction. Sugars provide calories without satiety, often leading to overconsumption of calories. Excess calories that are not used for energy are converted into fat and stored in the body, contributing to obesity. Over time, the constant demand for insulin can lead to insulin resistance, a precursor to type 2 diabetes. Sugars feed harmful bacteria in the mouth, leading to tooth decay and gum diseases. High sugar intake can increase the risk of heart disease by elevating blood pressure, inflammation, and triglyceride levels. According to the American Heart Association (AHA), men should consume no more than 9 teaspoons (36 grams or 150 calories) of added sugar per day; women should consume no more than 6 teaspoons (25 grams or 100 calories) per day.

HIGH-SUGAR FOODS TO LIMIT OR AVOID

- Baked goods, like cakes, cookies, donuts, and pastries
- Candy and other sweets
- Cereals and granola bars
- Dairy-based desserts like ice cream
- Fruit juices and sports drinks
- Specialty coffees and teas
- Sugar-sweetened beverages, like sodas
- Sweetened condiments and salad dressings
- Sweetened yogurts

NATURAL SUGARS

Natural sugars are still sugar in terms of the added and unnecessary calories they provide and should be limited. However, it's unfair to say they should be avoided altogether, as they do provide some nutritional benefits.

Agave syrup: Although high in fructose, agave syrup has a low glycemic index, so it doesn't spike blood sugar as quickly as table sugar. It's also sweeter than sugar, so you can use less to achieve the same level of sweetness.

Coconut sugar: Coconut sugar contains small amounts of minerals such as calcium, iron, potassium, and zinc as well as inulin, a type of fiber that may help improve gut health and slow glucose absorption.

Honey: Rich in antioxidants, antibacterial properties, and anti-inflammatory effects, honey also contains trace amounts of vitamins and minerals like vitamin C, calcium, and iron. Honey may also help with seasonal allergies, and it can soothe sore throats.

Maple syrup: Maple syrup, which contains antioxidants, zinc, calcium, potassium, and manganese, has a lower glycemic index compared to refined sugar, meaning it causes slower blood sugar spikes. Its natural sweetness can be used in moderation as a sugar substitute.

Molasses: A byproduct of sugarcane or sugar beet production, molasses is packed with iron, calcium, magnesium, potassium, and B vitamins. It also contains antioxidants and is often used to boost mineral intake, especially for those with iron deficiencies.

Reducing sugar doesn't mean giving up sweet flavor or enjoyment; instead:

1. **Choose unsweetened beverages.** Drink water, herbal teas, or coffee. For flavor, infuse water with slices of citrus fruit, strawberries, or cucumber.

2. **Cook and bake at home.** Prepare meals and baked goods at home so you control the sugar content. Spices such as cinnamon and vanilla can enhance

flavor without adding sugar, and adding bananas or applesauce adds sweetness and fiber.

3. **Opt for whole fruits.** Whole fruits, such as apples, berries, and oranges, provide natural sweetness along with antioxidants, fiber, and vitamins.

4. **Read labels.** When buying packaged foods, check the labels for "added sugars."

5. **Use artificial sweeteners.** Generally recognized as safe, non-nutritive sweeteners like stevia and Splenda provide calorie-free sweetness.

Please remember, we are simply limiting these added sugars, not strictly eliminating, fearing, or obsessing about them. You must promise me that you absolutely will have a piece of birthday cake on your birthday, okay?! The idea here is that we make an intentional effort to *reduce* our sugar consumption in an effort to prioritize more nutrient-dense foods instead. It's a shift toward less frequency and smaller portions, not a restriction.

Fiber

Fiber, a type of carbohydrate that the body cannot digest, is essential for maintaining good health. It comes in two types: soluble and insoluble. Soluble fiber dissolves in water to form a gel-like substance and helps lower blood cholesterol and glucose levels. Foods high in soluble fiber include oats, legumes, and fruits. Insoluble fiber adds bulk to stools and helps prevent constipation. Foods containing insoluble fiber are whole grains, vegetables, and nuts.

Adequate fiber intake is associated with a reduced risk of type 2 diabetes, heart disease, and certain cancers. It also promotes satiety, aiding in weight management. The Academy of Nutrition and Dietetics recommends consuming about 14 grams of fiber per every 1,000 calories consumed. The USDA provides general recommendations for fiber for adults as follows:

Men

- Ages 19 to 50: 31 to 34 grams per day
- Ages 51 and older: 28 grams per day

Women

- Ages 19 to 50: 25 to 28 grams per day
- Ages 51 and older: 22 grams per day

PREBIOTIC VS. PROBIOTIC FOODS VS. SUPPLEMENTS

Prebiotics and probiotics play distinct roles in maintaining gut health. Prebiotics are nondigestible fibers that feed beneficial gut bacteria, promoting a healthy microbiome to support digestion, vitamin and mineral absorption, and immune system function. Foods rich in prebiotics include bananas, garlic, Jerusalem artichokes, and onions. Unlike prebiotics, probiotics are live beneficial bacteria found in fermented foods such as kefir, kimchi, sauerkraut, and yogurt. They help maintain a balanced gut flora and can improve digestion and immune function. Although probiotic supplements are available—and it's important to choose reputable brands with verified bacterial strains—it's often preferable to obtain prebiotics and probiotics through foods, as they supply additional nutrients.

The term "gut health" has become a popular marketing buzzword, often used to sell probiotics, supplements, and various health products. To actually improve gut health, focus on consuming a diet rich in diverse, fiber-filled plant foods, including fruits, legumes, nuts, seeds, vegetables, and whole grains. Fermented foods, which naturally contain probiotics, can also support healthy gut flora. More important for overall gut health than any supplement are regular physical activity, adequate sleep, and managing stress. Additionally, avoiding excessive use of antibiotics, unless necessary, helps maintain the delicate balance of gut bacteria.

The average fiber intake for Americans falls significantly short of the recommended daily amounts. According to the National Health and Nutrition Examination Survey (NHANES) data, adult women typically consume 15 to 17 grams of fiber per day, whereas adult men average 17 to 19 grams per day.

What If Increasing Fiber Causes Discomfort?

On a GLP-1 medication, especially if feeling overly full, overloading fiber is likely a culprit for your gastrointestinal discomfort. Increasing fiber intake too quickly can cause issues such as bloating, cramping, or gas. To minimize these effects, gradually increase fiber-rich foods to allow your digestive system time to adjust. Drinking plenty of water is also helpful, as fiber needs water to move smoothly through the digestive tract.

FATS

Fats are tricky. They are a necessary component to a balanced nutrition plan yet often problematic, especially on GLP-1s. Dietary fats provide the densest source of energy among the macronutrients, with each gram of fat providing about 9 calories. Fats help with the absorption of fat-soluble vitamins (A, D, E, and K) and are vital for hormone production. See chapter 8 for more healthy fat options.

However, excessive consumption of certain types of fats can lead to excessive calorie intake, weight gain, and health issues. While on a GLP-1 medication, high-fat foods can strongly affect GI side effects and low appetite.

Balancing fat intake by choosing healthier options can improve overall health while still allowing you to enjoy flavorful foods. Here are some healthier alternatives:

1. Add avocado to your diet, a nutrient-rich fruit that provides healthy monounsaturated fats.

2. Choose healthy cooking oils rich in unsaturated fats, such as avocado oil, canola oil, or olive oil, to replace butter and margarine. Spray oil products can help control portion sizes.

3. Consume lean proteins, such as skinless poultry, fish, and plant-based proteins like beans, lentils, and tofu.

4. Cook meals at home to control the type and amount of fat used and consumed, and bake or grill foods instead of frying them to reduce overall fat content.

5. Enjoy nuts and seeds, such as almonds, chia seeds, flaxseed, and walnuts, in moderation, all excellent sources of healthy fats, vitamins, and minerals.

6. Substitute low-fat dairy or nonfat dairy products, such as yogurt, milk, and cheese, for their full-fat versions.

FOODS WITH HIGH AMOUNTS OF UNHEALTHY FATS

- Baked goods and pastries
- Fast foods
- Fatty cuts of meats, such as chicken thighs, short ribs, steak
- Fried foods
- Full-fat dairy products
- Margarine and shortening
- Processed meats, such as bacon and sausage
- Snack foods like potato chips

Unsaturated vs. Saturated Fats

Unsaturated fats are generally considered heart healthy and are found in plant-based oils (like canola, olive, and sunflower oils), nuts, seeds, avocado, and fatty fish. Unsaturated fats can be further divided into monounsaturated and polyunsaturated fats. Monounsaturated fats help reduce bad cholesterol levels, lowering the risk of heart disease and stroke. Polyunsaturated fats include omega-3 and omega-6 fatty acids, essential for brain function and cell growth, and should be obtained through your diet because the body cannot produce them.

Saturated fats, found primarily in animal products (such as meat and dairy) and some tropical oils (like coconut and palm oils), have been linked to increased levels of LDL ("bad") cholesterol and an elevated risk of heart disease. However, recent research suggests that the link between saturated fats and heart disease might not be as strong as once thought, reinforcing the importance of overall balanced dietary patterns and looking at foods more holistically rather than focusing on individual nutrients in isolation. While total elimination of saturated fats may not be necessary, we do see that people who eat a lot of these animal foods don't usually eat enough plants to compensate! Focusing on the healthy foods you can add is often more important than totally avoiding foods that may be less health promoting!

QUICK RECAP

- **Unhealthy fats** are saturated fats, such as those found in animal products.
- **Healthy fats** are unsaturated fats, such as those found in nuts and plant oils.
- **Both may make GLP-1 side effects worse and should be consumed in moderation.**
- Fats are high in calories, so portion size is important.
- Including fat in your nutrition plan can help keep you full and satisfied.

Caloric Density, Satiety, and Delayed Gastric Emptying

As you've learned, fats are the most calorically dense macronutrient, providing 9 calories per gram, more than twice the amount provided by carbohydrates or proteins. This high-caloric density means smaller amounts of fat can contribute significantly to daily caloric intake. While this makes it easier to consume excess calories if not monitored, fat's high energy content can be advantageous for those with high energy needs, such as athletes or those losing too much weight too quickly. Moreover, the caloric density of fats makes them a valuable component of a nutrition plan that provides satiety.

One of the most notable effects of dietary fats is their ability to promote satiety, that feeling of fullness after eating. Fats slow the digestive process and promote the release of satiety hormones such as leptin and peptide YY (PYY). Including healthy fats in meals can help reduce hunger and control appetite, making it easier to stick to recommended portion sizes and avoid unnecessary snacking. This satiety effect is particularly beneficial for weight management, as it can help prevent overeating and maintain a steady, balanced diet. So while I recommend keeping an eye on your portion sizes, I'm not saying healthy fats should be avoided altogether!

Dietary fats play a role in delaying gastric emptying, the process by which food leaves the stomach and enters the small intestine. By slowing gastric emptying, fats can enhance nutrient absorption and stabilize blood sugar levels, preventing rapid spikes and dips that can trigger hunger. Knowing that GLP-1 medications also delay gastric emptying, it is reasonable to see that overconsumption of dietary fats in combination with the medication can cause discomfort, side effects, and, ultimately, undereating.

THE IMPORTANCE OF PLANTS

In your journey toward weight loss and improved health, the significance of incorporating plants into your balanced diet—specifically fruits and vegetables—cannot be overstated.

Fruits are a gold mine of essential vitamins, minerals, and antioxidants. They are typically low in calories and high in fiber, which can help promote satiety and reduce overall caloric intake. Research has consistently linked fruit consumption with healthy body weight. Moreover, fruits are packed with vital nutrients. For instance, berries, such as blueberries and strawberries, contain anthocyanins, a type of antioxidant linked to reduced inflammation and improved cardiovascular health.

One prevalent myth surrounding fruits is that they should be avoided due to their sugar content. Although fruits do contain natural sugars, these are accompanied by fiber, which slows sugar absorption and prevents blood sugar spikes. In fact, people who consume more whole fruits have a lower risk of type 2 diabetes compared to those who do not. The health benefits of fruit outweigh the concerns when consumed as part of a balanced eating pattern. To maximize the benefits of fruits:

- Aim to fill half of your breakfast plate with a variety of fruits.
- Choose whole fruits over dried fruits, fruit juices, or smoothies.
- Prioritize variety—all fruits bring different nutrient profiles, and no fruits are better than others, just different.
- Use fruits in snacks or desserts, paired with protein.

And just like fruits, vegetables are also an integral component of a weight loss–friendly nutrition plan. They are nutrient-dense and usually low in calories. Eating a variety of vegetables is linked to lower levels of obesity and improved overall health due to their role in decreasing inflammation, enhancing digestion, and providing antioxidants. Most research finds that increasing vegetable intake is correlated with a reduction in body weight and fat mass. To effectively include more vegetables in your diet:

- Experiment with different cooking techniques—grilling, roasting, or steaming can enhance flavors. Roasting can caramelize vegetables' natural sugars, increasing appeal and palatability.
- Hide vegetables by blending them into foods like pasta sauces, muffins, and ground meats.
- Keep cut veggies on hand for quick snacking or cooking.
- Season and sauce your veggies for more flavor. A little bit of ranch doesn't offset the benefits; in fact, the fats in ranch dressing can increase vitamin absorption!

FRESH VS. FROZEN VS. CANNED

The debate about the differences and benefits among fresh, frozen, and canned fruits and vegetables only decreases the ease with which folks can eat more produce! Fresh produce is often perceived as the healthiest option but (maybe surprisingly) can actually contain fewer nutrients if not consumed promptly. Frozen fruits and vegetables are typically picked at their peak ripeness and flash frozen, preserving many of their nutrients. Canned vegetables can be convenient and affordable. Look for fruits packed in 100 percent fruit juice and choose "low-sodium" varieties of beans, fruits, and vegetables.

LOCAL VS. ORGANIC VS. CONVENTIONAL

Choosing between local, organic, and conventional produce presents a nuanced choice. Locally sourced fruits and vegetables might be fresher and support local economies. Organic options are grown without *synthetic* pesticides and fertilizers, improving environmental sustainability and reducing chemical exposure, but the perception that organic food is always healthier can lead to increased costs and reduced overall consumption of fruits and vegetables. Consider joining a local CSA program for access to local and organic produce at reasonable prices. This promotes sustainability and supports local farming efforts while providing fresh seasonal produce. However, when it comes to nutrient content, the differences are minimal and conventional produce often provides the same (or better) nutritional value than the organic counterpart for a variety of reasons, despite the general (incorrect) assumption that organic is more nutritious. Benefits of conventional farming practices include:

1. **Use of synthetic fertilizers:** Conventional farming often relies on synthetic fertilizers that provide crops with high levels of essential nutrients like nitrogen, phosphorus, and potassium. This can lead to faster growth and potentially higher concentrations of certain nutrients in the plants compared to organic crops, which rely on natural fertilizers like compost or manure.

2. **Pest and disease control:** Conventional farming allows the use of a wide range of chemical pesticides and herbicides, which can lead to healthier plants that are less stressed. Reduced stress from pests and disease may allow

plants to allocate more energy to growth and nutrient accumulation, whereas organic crops may experience more pest pressure, which could affect their nutrient composition.

3. **Controlled growing environment:** Conventional farming techniques allow for more controlled environmental conditions, which can lead to more consistent nutrient profiles across produce. Organic farming, especially on small-scale farms, may be more susceptible to environmental stress.

However, it is important to note that the big picture difference in nutrition between organic and conventional produce tends to be very small, and factors like post-harvest handling can play a larger role in nutritional differences.

And please, do yourself a favor: just ignore the Environmental Working Group's (EWG) "Dirty Dozen" list, which highlights fruits and vegetables with the highest pesticide residue; it creates an exaggerated perception of risk associated with conventionally grown produce, fostering a totally unnecessary fear of pesticides while overlooking the broader context of their safety. Remember, it's the dose that makes the poison. A woman could consume the equivalent of all the pesticide residue from 13,225 servings of blueberries (#11 on EWG's 2024 Dirty Dozen list) in one day without any negative effect—even if the blueberries have the highest pesticide residue recorded for blueberries by USDA. You can check the risk of other foods you may be concerned about using the Pesticide Residue Calculator on the website SafeFruitsandVeggies.com/pesticide-residue-calculator/ provided by the Alliance for Food and Farming (AFF), a nonprofit organization formed in 1989 that represents both organic and conventional farmers of fruits and vegetables. It is of course okay to have a preference for organic produce if you can afford it, but please make that choice for some other reason than fear.

A NOTE ON HIGH-SODIUM FOODS

Sodium, an essential mineral, is key in maintaining fluid balance, contracting muscles, and transmitting nerve impulses. However, excess sodium can be harmful. The recommended daily sodium intake for healthy adults is less than 2,300 milligrams, equivalent to about 1 teaspoon of salt. For people with high blood pressure, the recommendation is to further reduce sodium intake to 1,500 milligrams per day.

Sodium attracts and holds water, which can increase blood volume. Elevated blood volume forces the heart to work harder, creating pressure in the arteries, thereby increasing blood pressure. Chronic high blood pressure can damage blood vessels, leading to heart disease, stroke, and kidney problems. The kidneys regulate fluid balance by filtering out excess sodium, but high sodium intake can overload unhealthy kidneys, further impairing kidney function. High sodium levels can also cause calcium to be excreted in the urine, which may lead to decreased bone density and an increased risk of osteoporosis over time.

High-sodium foods are abundant in the modern diet, particularly in processed and restaurant foods. Common examples include:

- Bread and bakery products
- Canned soups and vegetables
- Cheese and dairy products
- Frozen meals and instant foods
- Processed meats such as bacon, deli meats, ham, and sausages
- Sauces and condiments
- Processed snack foods such as chips and crackers

Many of the same strategies and alternatives you've learned so far (hint: balance, portion control, prioritizing whole foods) apply to controlling sodium intake. Additionally, you can drain and rinse canned foods to remove some of the sodium present; choose fresh foods over processed or opt for frozen versions of fresh whole foods; use herbs, spices, and citrus to flavor foods instead of salt; and choose low-sodium products and low-sodium menu items when eating out.

ULTRA-PROCESSED FOODS

In our busy lives, processed and convenience foods have integrated seamlessly into our daily diets (with plenty of benefits), yet a particular category of these foods draws increasing scrutiny: ultra-processed foods. Ultra-processed foods are significantly altered from their original form through industrial processes and typically contain substances not commonly used in home cooking, such as artificial flavors, colors, emulsifiers, preservatives, and other additives. Common examples include sugary drinks, packaged snacks, candies, instant noodles, soups, processed meats, ready-made meals, and even some types of bread. While ultra-processed foods offer convenience, and sometimes affordability, they pose several health hazards when consumed in excess.

One primary concern regarding ultra-processed foods is their impact on nutrient balance; they contain high levels of sugar, unhealthy fats, and salt, yet lack essential nutrients such as fiber, minerals, and vitamins. The combination of sugar, fat, and salt can render these foods highly palatable, leading to overeating and contributing to weight gain that may promote metabolic dysfunction. Lacking necessary fiber and containing additives that may disrupt the gut microbiome, these foods can also lead to digestive irregularities and dysbiosis. While correlation is not causation, it is certainly a strong enough association to be cautious.

Despite their significant drawbacks, ultra-processed foods do offer some benefits. For individuals with busy lifestyles who lack the time to prepare fresh meals from scratch, ultra-processed foods provide a quick and easy meal solution, and they're often cheaper than healthier, whole food options, making them an economically viable source of caloric intake for individuals with limited financial resources. Their long shelf life helps reduce food waste and provides reliable food sources in regions with limited access to fresh produce. In emergency situations or disaster-relief scenarios, ultra-processed foods can serve as a readily available and durable source of nutrition when other food options are scarce. Some ultra-processed foods are fortified with vitamins and minerals, addressing specific nutrient deficiencies in certain populations. And although ultra-processed foods can be convenient and useful in specific instances, their consumption should be balanced with whole, unprocessed foods to ensure good overall nutrition. Indulging occasionally in your favorite treats is perfectly normal and can be part of a healthy lifestyle.

LET'S TALK ABOUT POOP

Your bowel movements can provide valuable insights into your overall health status, as variations in stool color, frequency, consistency, and odor can indicate different aspects of digestive health. A healthy bowel movement is typically brown, due to the presence of bile, and should be well formed but not too hard or too loose. The frequency of bowel movements can vary from person to person, but it is generally considered healthy to have between three a day to three a week. Daily bowel movements are actually incredibly rare! It's also very normal for bowel movement size and frequency to decrease when taking a GLP-1 medication as a result of the delayed gastric emptying and decreased volume of foods consumed.

It's also smart to monitor for changes in stool color and alert your providers; black or red can indicate bleeding in the digestive tract, whereas pale stools might suggest issues with bile flow. These things are super rare but should not be ignored!

Similarly, persistent foul odors could point to malabsorption issues or infections. Paying attention to these characteristics can help you identify potential health concerns early and seek medical advice when necessary to maintain optimal digestive function and overall health.

LET'S TALK ABOUT HYDRATION

I can't tell you how many people report that the reason they didn't lose weight might be because they didn't drink enough water that week. I'm sorry if this bursts your bubble (See what I did there with the pun?), but while *adequate* hydration is important for many health reasons, there is no direct correlation between more hydration and more weight loss. There is some truth to the idea that the *habit* of drinking more fluids can decrease overall food intake or increase awareness of other healthy habits. But, in a world full of very fancy reusable tumblers, folks are sometimes drinking excessive amounts of fluids. The fact is, our body knows exactly how much water it needs and will expel the excess! Aiming for 64 to 82 ounces (1.9 to 2.4 L) per day is *plenty*.

On a GLP-1 medication, it is important to be more intentional about hydration, but that doesn't mean you need more than the average Joe. GLP-1s can decrease the sensation of thirst in the same way it suppresses appetite, increasing the risk for dehydration. We also forget how much hydration we get from foods—and if we are eating less, we may need to drink a little more.

If you're dealing with side effects, especially vomiting or diarrhea, it is essential to replace these lost fluids to protect your kidneys. But drowning yourself in gallons per day is unnecessary. As long as you have light-colored urine, moist-feeling mouth, skin, and eyes, and are not fatigued, you're probably drinking enough.

Although water is probably the most important beverage for hydration, other options include coffee, diet beverages, herbal teas, sparkling water, unsweetened teas, and any other zero-calorie liquid.

ELECTROLYTES

Electrolyte supplements and drinks can be beneficial for folks on GLP-1 medications who are dealing with side effects, very low appetites, and fatigue or those who engage in high-intensity exercise. Electrolyte drinks can improve hydration levels during and after exercise, especially in prolonged activity or in hot environments. They can help restore electrolyte balance after intense workouts or illnesses (such as vomiting or diarrhea). However, use these products with caution. Many electrolyte drinks contain high levels of sugar that can counteract weight loss efforts. Excessive intake of electrolytes, like the amounts found in concentrated supplements, particularly sodium and potassium, can result in imbalances and lead to health issues such as hypertension or heart problems, especially for those with kidney disease.

THE MICRONUTRIENTS

Micronutrients—vitamins and minerals—are critical components of our diet that, although required in small amounts, play important roles in maintaining our health, supporting bodily functions, and preventing chronic diseases. Of course, we get the majority of vitamins and minerals via the foods we eat. Variety, adequacy, and balance are key, but when on a weight loss journey and limiting intakes, it's reasonable to worry that we may come up short in some areas, and supplements can be beneficial.

SUPPLEMENTS TO CONSIDER

To be clear, there are no *required* dietary supplements you need to take while on a GLP-1 medication. A balanced diet is the best source of essential nutrients, but some supplements are generally recognized as safe and useful, especially when dietary intake falls short or if you are losing weight too quickly. If you are concerned that you are deficient, consider asking your primary care provider for labs or working with your dietitian to evaluate your usual intakes and look for opportunities for improvement. If you're thinking about adding some supplements, these are the ones I think are worthwhile to consider, depending on your individual needs:

> **Calcium:** Essential for bone health, calcium can be lacking in diets, especially if you avoid dairy. Calcium carbonate and calcium citrate are common supplemental forms, with citrate being more easily absorbed on an empty stomach. Most adults need about 1,000 mg a day from both supplemental and food sources combined. The sweet spot for absorption is 500 mg. Do *not* take at the same time as a supplement containing iron.

> **Iron:** Particularly important for menstruating women, vegetarians, and individuals with anemia, iron supplements help with oxygen transport and energy levels. However, iron should generally be taken under medical supervision due to its risks of toxicity. Adult males need 8 mg a day; most adult women need 18 mg (27 mg in pregnancy) from both food and supplements. It's common for iron supplements to contribute to constipation, but taking this *every other day* instead of daily can help. Avoid taking with dairy foods or calcium

PRO TIP

Every individual's supplementation plan should be truly individualized based on their unique needs. If someone is recommending a "protocol" just because you're on a weight loss journey or taking a GLP-1 medication, I'd venture to guess they are just trying to make money. Remember, more is not always better (sometimes actually harmful), and more cost doesn't always provide more benefits. Unless you have a known deficiency or medical need, when it comes to supplements, my overarching point of view is something like this: If you feel it helps you, and there aren't any known risks, and you like using it and can afford it, then it's probably fine, but you also probably don't need it.

supplements. Tea, coffee, and sodas can also inhibit absorption. Vitamin C drinks and foods (orange juice, fruit) can improve absorption.

Magnesium: This mineral is involved in more than three hundred biochemical reactions in the body, including muscle function, nerve function, and blood sugar regulation. Magnesium supplements can be particularly beneficial if your diet is low in magnesium-rich foods like nuts and leafy greens. Of course there are several different types of magnesium with slightly different benefits, but generally speaking, adults need about 300 to 400 mg of elemental magnesium per day from all sources. Caution if you struggle with loose stools—magnesium can make this worse.

Multivitamins: A daily multivitamin can help fill nutritional gaps, especially for those with restricted diets or increased nutritional needs. To determine if a multivitamin is "complete," check the label for essential vitamins and minerals that meet your nutritional needs. A complete multivitamin typically includes a broad spectrum of vitamins (A, C, D, E, K, and all B vitamins) and important minerals like calcium, magnesium, zinc, and iron. It should provide close to 100 percent of the dietary reference intake (DRI) for most of these nutrients. Additionally, make sure the multivitamin matches your age, gender, and health goals, as certain formulations are designed for specific groups. Be wary of any labels with 200 percent-plus of any particular component! More than the recommended daily value is not always better—it could actually be harmful!

Omega-3 fatty acids: Found in fish oil or algae oil supplements, omega-3s contribute to brain function, heart health, and reducing inflammation. Eicosapentaenoic acid (EPA) and docosahexaenoic acid (DHA) are considered the most beneficial forms of omega-3 fatty acids because of their significant health benefits and bioavailability. EPA is known for its anti-inflammatory properties and DHA is crucial for brain and eye health, particularly in fetal development and throughout life. Both EPA and DHA are found in fatty fish and are more readily absorbed and utilized by the body compared to other omega-3 forms, such as alpha-linolenic acid (ALA), which is less efficiently processed in the body. There aren't very clear guidelines for exactly *how much* omega-3 should be supplemented, but common fish oil products offer about 500 mg to 1,000 mg per day.

Vitamin D: Many people, particularly those living in northern latitudes or with limited sun exposure, may not get enough vitamin D, which supports bone health, immune function, and mood regulation. For its superior bioavailability, the recommended supplement form is vitamin D3 (cholecalciferol). While the RDA is only 400 IU, supplementation of about 1,000 IU to 2,000 IU daily helps replenish low levels. It's important to know that very high doses of vitamin D can

PRO TIP

Let's be clear: Any "natural" supplements claiming to provide the same benefits as GLP-1 medications are a scam. GLP-1 medications are rigorously tested, standardized, and approved by regulatory bodies, providing a level of safety and efficacy that most natural alternatives cannot match. If berberine or probiotics produced the same results, big pharma would have cashed in on that decades ago.

be harmful, so you should never take any supplements with more than 4,000 IU of vitamin D unless recommended by a physician.

Vitamin B 12: If you're vegan or vegetarian, I do recommend a daily B 12 supplement (or at least a multivitamin that contains B 12) at the RDA of 2.4 mcg per day. People on metformin or those who take a lot of acid-suppressing medications for reflux should also supplement with B 12. Fun fact: Most B 12 supplements have excessive levels of this vitamin because it is water soluble; more isn't better—you're just gonna pee it out! The idea that B 12 will help with fatigue or energy is not well supported. Instead of adding a supplement for fatigue, I'd add carbs and water first.

BONUS SUPPLEMENT

Creatine: Creatine, a popular and safe supplement known for its benefits in enhancing athletic performance and muscle growth, works by increasing the availability of adenosine triphosphate (ATP), the energy currency of cells, which can improve strength, power, and high-intensity exercise performance. It supports faster post-exercise recovery, reduces muscle cell damage and inflammation, and can increase muscle mass when combined with resistance training. Beyond sports, emerging research suggests potential cognitive benefits, such as improved memory and mental fatigue resistance. The recommended dosing of creatine monohydrate is 5 grams a day—take every day whether or not it's a workout day. Best taken in the morning, as it can impact sleep if taken late in the evening. You may notice a two- to three-pound (1 to 1.4 kg) weight gain from water weight after starting creatine (resulting in bigger-looking muscles), but this is nothing to worry about!

A NOTE ON BARIATRIC SURGERY

It is extremely important to continue to take your bariatric multivitamins for the rest of your life and to regularly check in with your primary care provider or bariatric surgeon to check vitamin and mineral levels.

Recommendations for supplementation from The American Society for Metabolic and Bariatric Surgery (ASMBS) are as follows. Recommendations for the vertical sleeve gastrectomy (VSG) and Roux-en-Y gastric bypass (RYGB) are the same unless otherwise stated:

- Calcium: 1,200 to 1,500 mg per day, in 2 or 3 doses (separate from iron); calcium citrate is better absorbed for RYGB; carbonate is cheaper and okay for VSG

- Copper*: 100 percent of recommended dietary allowance (RDA) in the multivitamin (increase to 200 percent for RYGB)

- Fat-soluble vitamins A, E, and K: Recommended dietary allowance via multivitamin

- Folic acid: 400 to 800 mcg via multivitamin; 800 to 1,000 mg if childbearing potential

- Iron: Men or postmenopausal individuals, 18 mg per day; if menstruating, 45 to 60 mg per day; taken separate from calcium supplements

- Thiamine: 12 mg via multivitamin, additional 50 mg via B-complex

- Vitamin B12: oral 300 to 500 mcg per day

- Vitamin D3: 3,000 IU per day

- Zinc: 100 percent of RDA (*Zinc to copper ratio of 8:1 to prevent copper deficiency)

CHOOSING A QUALITY SUPPLEMENT

Not all supplements are created equal. To choose a quality product:

- Check for third-party testing: Supplements tested by independent organizations like the US Pharmacopeia (USP), ConsumerLab, or NSF International carry certifications ensuring the product contains what it claims without harmful contaminants.

- Consider bioavailability: Some forms of vitamins and minerals are better absorbed by the body. For example, magnesium citrate and glycinate are more bioavailable than magnesium oxide.

- Research the manufacturer: Reputable companies follow Good Manufacturing Practice (GMP) regulations and engage in transparent business practices, providing detailed information about ingredient sourcing and quality control.

Not all supplements live up to their hype, and most are probably a waste of money for minimal proven benefit, such as:

- Collagen supplements: Collagen is essential for skin, joint, and bone health, but the scientific evidence supporting the benefits of collagen supplements is still limited and not robustly conclusive.

- "Detox" supplements: The body has natural detoxification systems—primarily the liver and kidneys—that effectively eliminate toxins. Most detox supplements lack scientific backing and can be harmful alongside some medications.

- Excessive antioxidants: Supplements like high-dose vitamin C or E may sound beneficial, but excessive intake can potentially increase the risk of certain cancers and other health issues.

- Expensive multivitamins: High-priced multivitamins often don't provide better absorption or additional benefits compared to more reasonably priced options that meet RDA guidelines.

- Fat burners: These supplements often contain stimulants and other compounds that lack substantial evidence for weight loss and can have harmful side effects, including increased heart rate and blood pressure.

- Homeopathic remedies: Homeopathy is based on highly diluted substances that theoretically stimulate the body's healing processes. However, scientific research shows that these remedies generally lack efficacy beyond a placebo effect.

OTHER NUTRITIONAL CONSIDERATIONS

So, we've covered the macro and micro nutrients in detail and yet, there's still so much more **stuff** that we consume as part of our usual dietary patterns. Thanks to modern science and technology, many foods have been manufactured in a way that they contain artificial sweeteners or preservatives. While generally safe, and very unlikely to be a major contributor in your health and weight loss journey, they are worth exploring in more detail. Here we will also learn more about caffeine and alcohol, especially as they may be more relevant to your GLP-1 medication experience.

ARTIFICIAL SWEETENERS

Artificial sweeteners, like aspartame, stevia, and sucralose, are immensely popular for reducing caloric intake without sacrificing sweetness. Although effective for satisfying a sweet craving, their long-term health effects remain a subject of debate. While the FDA has classified many artificial sweeteners as safe, individual sensitivities and emerging studies call for more research on their long-term effects, particularly concerning gut health and metabolic processes. Sugar alcohols, like erythritol, tend to upset sensitive stomachs. You know we've all had one of those fake ice cream pints (looking at you Halo Top) that didn't "sit well." Moderation is key; using these sweeteners occasionally and not as a primary source of sweetness may be the best approach. Best believe I will continue to have a few crisp Diet Cokes per week, especially while losing weight, and especially as a substitute for a sugar-sweetened alternative.

PRESERVATIVES

Common food preservatives and additives, such as sodium benzoate, citric acid, and nitrates, play a significant role in modern food systems by extending shelf life, preventing spoilage, and enhancing flavor. Sodium benzoate and potassium sorbate, for example, inhibit bacterial and fungal growth, while citric acid acts as a preservative and flavor enhancer in beverages and processed foods. Nitrates are often used in cured meats to preserve color and prevent the growth of harmful bacteria like *Clostridium botulinum*. These additives are generally recognized as safe (GRAS) by regulatory bodies like the FDA when consumed in typical amounts. However, some are controversial due to potential health concerns.

For example, nitrates, when consumed in very large quantities or converted into nitrosamines during cooking, have been linked to cancer risk. Similarly, some artificial colors and flavors are associated with allergic reactions or hyperactivity in sensitive individuals. It's important to remember that any potential risk increases with increased exposure. So, keeping portion sizes of processed foods to moderate levels and increasing your intake of whole foods can help protect you from any theoretical (yet unproved) concerns.

ALCOHOL

In the context of weight loss, alcohol contains calories we just don't need, providing energy without essential nutrients—and these calories add up quickly, making it easy to exceed daily limits. Moreover, alcohol can impair our judgment, often leading to poor dietary choices, like the Taco Bell drive-thru at 2 a.m. Chronic alcohol use can lead to nutritional deficiencies, as it interferes with the absorption of vital vitamins and minerals, particularly vitamin A, B vitamins, and magnesium. Alcohol can negatively affect liver function, increasing the risk of liver diseases such as fatty liver, hepatitis, and cirrhosis. It also has a detrimental effect on mental health, contributing to anxiety, depression, and cognitive impairments. Excessive alcohol intake can disrupt sleep patterns, which can further exacerbate health issues.

It is essential to approach alcohol mindfully, understanding the balance between enjoyment and health risks. Anecdotal reports from patients show that GLP-1 medications may help individuals experience fewer cravings for alcohol, particularly in situations where emotional or environmental triggers would typically lead to excessive drinking. *And, rumor has it, the hangovers are way worse!* If you are struggling to decrease your alcohol intake, seeking help is an important step toward recovery.

It's also important to let your prescriber know if you are currently struggling with excess alcohol intake prior to starting your medication. GLP-1 medications can reduce your ability to tolerate or even crave alcohol (yay); however, a rapid

PRO TIP

While there is no proven health benefit to alcohol that outweighs the risk, we do have some guidelines for how much alcohol we can consume to minimize harm. The Dietary Guidelines for alcohol intake suggest that if alcohol is consumed, it should be done in moderation, which is defined as up to one drink per day for women and up to two drinks per day for men. A standard drink is generally considered to be:

- 12 ounces (355 ml) of beer (about 5 percent alcohol)
- 5 ounces (150 ml) of wine (about 12 percent alcohol)
- 1.5 ounces (45 ml) of distilled spirits (about 40 percent alcohol)

Unlike some medications that have warning labels related to alcohol, GLP-1s do not. Excess alcohol intake can increase your risk for pancreatitis, a rare but known complication of GLP-1 medications, so combining the two could be problematic. So what's my recommendation here? A margarita on a beach vacation, a glass of wine at an anniversary party, or a flute of champagne at New Year's is probably fine! Daily use or weekend binges? Not advised.

decrease in alcohol intake after regular use can lead to withdrawal, which can be dangerous and require medical support.

CAFFEINE

Caffeine, found in coffee, tea, and energy drinks, is one of the most widely consumed psychoactive substances in the world. Up to 400 milligrams (mg) of caffeine a day appears to be safe for most healthy adults (that's about 4 cups, or 950 ml, of coffee). Its stimulating effects can enhance alertness and concentration, but it also plays a role in metabolism. Caffeine has been shown to temporarily boost metabolism and enhance fat oxidation and may aid in appetite suppression for a short period. However, your tolerance to caffeine should be balanced against its potential to disrupt sleep patterns and cause anxiety. A quick reminder: Coffee is not a meal. And, if you are struggling with reflux on your GLP-1 medication, coffee may be to blame (especially if taken with cream). You may also find that your sleep is more affected in the evenings if you take in caffeine later in the day, thanks to the delayed gastric emptying. Generally speaking, occasional intake of diet sodas, energy drinks, and fancy coffee is totally fine, especially if it helps you get through a busy day—but be honest with yourself and check in on your limits! Too much of a good thing is still too much!

THE SCIENCE BEHIND NUTRITION FACTS AND FOOD LABELING

Now that you know what you're going to prioritize while making food choices, understanding how to read nutrition labels is going to be an indispensable skill for making informed nutrition choices. With our current state of misinformation and sketchy marketing tactics, this can feel like a daunting task, but I hope to provide the facts on how these labels work, so you can know what's worth paying attention to and what's just noise.

The history of the Nutrition Facts label in the United States is a product of growing public interest in health and nutrition, combined with a series of legislative measures aimed at improving consumer awareness. This label was designed to provide clear, consistent information about the nutritional content of foods, helping consumers make informed dietary choices. The FDA established specific guidelines for the label, outlining key components such as serving sizes, calorie counts, and nutrient measurements (including fats, carbohydrates, and proteins), with the purpose of enhancing the public's understanding of nutrition.

Regulations governing the claims that food companies can make on their product labels are primarily established by the US Food and Drug Administration (FDA) and the Federal Trade Commission (FTC) in the United States. These regulations are intended to prevent misleading information and ensure consumers receive accurate, truthful information regarding the nutritional and health attributes of food products. But keep in mind, nutrition labels can sometimes be misleading. Manufacturers may use smaller serving sizes to make the nutritional content appear healthier. Additionally, sugars can be listed under various names like high fructose corn syrup, dextrose, and sucrose, making it challenging to recognize hidden sugars.

GLP-1 Label Reading Priorities

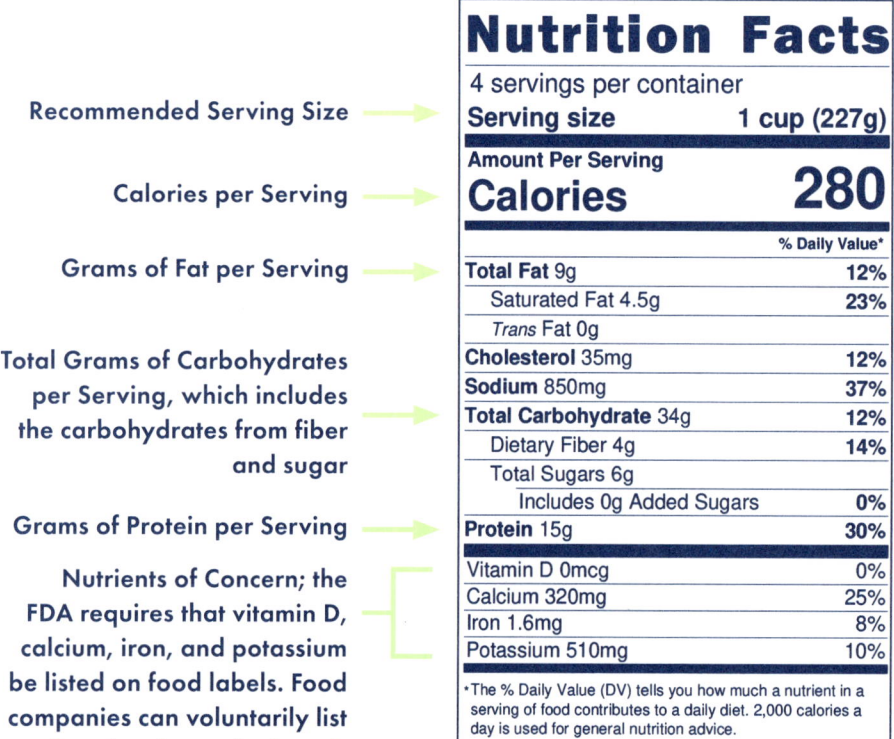

Recommended Serving Size →

Calories per Serving →

Grams of Fat per Serving →

Total Grams of Carbohydrates per Serving, which includes the carbohydrates from fiber and sugar →

Grams of Protein per Serving →

Nutrients of Concern; the FDA requires that vitamin D, calcium, iron, and potassium be listed on food labels. Food companies can voluntarily list other vitamins and minerals on the label

Nutrition Facts

4 servings per container

Serving size	1 cup (227g)

Amount Per Serving

Calories	280

	% Daily Value*
Total Fat 9g	12%
Saturated Fat 4.5g	23%
Trans Fat 0g	
Cholesterol 35mg	12%
Sodium 850mg	37%
Total Carbohydrate 34g	12%
Dietary Fiber 4g	14%
Total Sugars 6g	
Includes 0g Added Sugars	0%
Protein 15g	30%
Vitamin D 0mcg	0%
Calcium 320mg	25%
Iron 1.6mg	8%
Potassium 510mg	10%

*The % Daily Value (DV) tells you how much a nutrient in a serving of food contributes to a daily diet. 2,000 calories a day is used for general nutrition advice.

You should also take a peek at the ingredients, which are listed in descending order of predominance by weight

Label Claims

Under the Nutrition Labeling and Education Act (NLEA) of 1990, a comprehensive framework was created to delineate specific categories of claims, including health claims, nutrient content claims, and structure/function claims. Claims such as "low-fat," "light," or "natural" do not always equal healthier options. It's essential to scrutinize these claims and read the ingredients list to make informed choices.

Health Claims

Health claims specifically link a food substance with a reduced risk of a disease or health-related condition. For example, a product may claim that "diets low in saturated fat and cholesterol may reduce the risk of coronary heart disease." However, for such claims to be made, they must meet stringent criteria, often based on scientific evidence reviewed by the FDA. This includes being supported by a significant body of scientific research, which the FDA evaluates before allowing these claims to appear on packaging.

Nutrient Claims

Nutrient content claims describe the level of a nutrient in a food product and are highly regulated as well. Common examples include terms like "low fat," "high fiber," or "sugar-free." To use these terms, food products must meet specific definitions set forth by the FDA. For instance, for a product to be labeled as "low fat," it must contain 3 grams of fat per serving or fewer, and "high fiber" requires at least 5 grams of fiber per serving.

Structure and Function Claims

These claims describe the role of a nutrient or ingredient in maintaining normal bodily functions but are not permitted to imply a connection to the prevention, treatment, or cure of a specific disease. For example, a product may state "Calcium helps build strong bones," providing consumers with information about how a product can contribute to overall health.

ORGANIC, NATURAL, AND NON-GMO

Another area of confusion lies in understanding the labels "organic," "natural," and "non-GMO." These terms actually relate to production methods rather than nutritional content but are often mistaken for indicators of nutritional superiority.

Organic

Organic foods are produced without synthetic pesticides, hormones, and antibiotics, which might result in lower levels of certain contaminants. However, scientific studies indicate that the nutritional content of organic foods is not significantly different from conventionally grown foods.

Natural

The term "natural" is even murkier, as it is not strictly regulated and can mean different things depending on the context. Generally, it suggests the absence of artificial ingredients or preservatives, but it does not guarantee that the product is lower in calories, sugars, or fats.

Non-GMO

Similarly, non-GMO foods are those that have not been genetically modified, but this label does not necessarily imply higher nutrition. The decision to consume non-GMO foods often hinges on ethical or environmental considerations rather than nutritional benefits. In the United States, genetically modified organisms (GMOs) primarily include a limited number of crops that have been engineered for specific traits, such as increased resistance to pests, herbicides, and environmental conditions. The most commonly grown GMO crops include canola, corn, cotton, and soybeans, with a significant portion of these being used for animal feed, processed foods, and biofuels. Although public perception often associates GMOs with health risks, a substantial body of scientific research indicates that GMOs are safe for human consumption and present numerous benefits. Genetically modified crops can produce higher yields, which support food security by making it possible to produce more food on less land. They also reduce the need for chemical pesticides, thereby benefiting the environment by decreasing agricultural runoff and promoting more sustainable farming practices. The enhanced resistance to pests and diseases can also result in lower food costs for consumers and farmers alike.

CHAPTER 07

PUTTING WHAT YOU KNOW INTO REAL-LIFE PRACTICE

E ating well is about so much more than what we eat. Sometimes the how—the behaviors, skills, and real-life practicalities and our mindset—can matter more! In this chapter, I want to help you explore and consider all the ways you can get food on your plate efficiently and enjoyably. When eating well becomes "just something you do well," not a chore, we know it'll last! In this chapter, we will discuss how to build motivation, achieve goals, and overcome challenges. You should walk away feeling empowered and prepared with a new library of skill for any situation in which this whole weight loss thing gets hard!

Motivation isn't something you just have—it's something you develop. It takes practice and self-assessment to build within your mind. At its core, motivation involves a dynamic interplay between intrinsic and extrinsic factors. Intrinsic motivation is driven by internal rewards and personal satisfaction, such as the desire to feel healthier or achieve a sense of accomplishment. Extrinsic motivation, on the other hand, stems from external rewards or pressures, like fitting into a particular dress size or receiving praise from others. Neuroscientific studies reveal that motivation is closely linked to the brain's reward system, involving neurotransmitters like dopamine, which play a significant role in pleasure and goal-setting behaviors.

GOAL SETTING

Weight loss and health changes can often seem like daunting challenges. Many embark on this journey with grand visions of rapid transformation, only to become discouraged when the results don't match their expectations. Understanding the science behind setting goals for weight loss can help you approach this journey in a more sustainable and realistic way, increasing your chances of long-term success.

Setting goals is key for any significant change, and weight loss is no exception. Goals provide direction and a clear target to aim for, breaking down what can seem like an overwhelming task into manageable, achievable steps. They transform abstract intentions into actionable plans. One of the first steps in setting effective weight loss goals is ensuring they are realistic and sustainable. Goals that are too ambitious can lead to frustration and burnout, whereas those that are too easy won't push you to make meaningful progress or change. The key is to find a balance.

Realistic goals are those that are achievable given your current lifestyle, commitments, and physical health. An example of a realistic weight loss goal might be aiming to lose 1 to 2 pounds (454 to 907 g) per week; gradual weight loss is more sustainable and healthier for the body. Sustainable goals are those that can be maintained over the long term. Instead of drastic measures that promise quick results, focus on changes you can integrate into your daily life.

Achievable goals help maintain motivation. As you consistently achieve your smaller goals, you build confidence and momentum that propel you toward your larger target. Celebrating these small victories can provide the encouragement needed to keep going. Sustainable changes are also more beneficial for your health. Rapid weight loss can lead to muscle loss, nutritional deficiencies, and a decreased metabolic rate, making it harder to maintain weight loss in the long term. Gradual, steady weight loss typically involves lifestyle changes, such as eating a healthier diet and getting regular physical activity, that improve overall health. By setting realistic and sustainable goals, you're less likely to feel overwhelmed and more able to continue your healthy habits over time.

SMART GOALS

A well-known method for setting effective goals is the SMART method, which stands for specific, measurable, achievable, relevant, and time-bound. This framework helps ensure your goals are clear and attainable.

- **Specific:** Goals should be clear and specific. Instead of saying, "I want to lose weight," specify how much weight you want to lose and by what means. For example, "I want to lose 10 pounds (4.5 kg) in three months by exercising three times a week and reducing my caloric intake by 500 calories per day."

- **Measurable:** Having measurable goals means you can track your progress. This could involve weekly weigh-ins or keeping a food diary. Tracking your progress helps you stay accountable to see how far you've come.

- **Achievable:** Goals should be challenging but attainable. Consider your current circumstances and set a target that pushes you without being impossible to achieve. It's important to stretch yourself a bit, but not so much that you set yourself up for failure.

- **Relevant:** Ensure your goals align with your broader objectives and values. Weight loss that aligns with your desire to improve overall health, participate in activities you enjoy, or increase your energy levels will be more meaningful and motivating.

- **Time-bound:** Setting a time frame for your goals creates urgency and accountability and helps you focus your efforts. A time-bound goal gives you a clear endpoint to work toward, which can help motivate you to stay on track.

Of course, it's important to periodically reassess your goals and adjust as needed. Life circumstances can change, and your initial goals might need to be modified. Be flexible and open to changing your strategy while staying committed to your overall objective.

AN ALTERNATIVE APPROACH: FAST GOALS

Although SMART goals are widely utilized, another effective approach to goal-setting is the FAST method, which stands for frequent, ambitious, specific, and transparent. FAST goals focus on maintaining momentum and accountability through frequent check-ins and ambitious targets that push you beyond your comfort zone. They are specific enough to provide clear direction and transparent in a way that allows for public sharing of progress, fostering a sense of communal support and responsibility. For example, setting a FAST goal might involve publicly sharing your aspiration to run a 5K in six months, with regular updates on social media about your progress. This method leverages both personal ambition and social accountability, which can be powerful motivators in your weight loss journey.

The ambitious nature and frequent reassessment of FAST goals align well with a growth mindset, which is the belief that abilities and health can be improved with effort and persistence. When individuals regularly review their progress and make necessary adjustments, they are more likely to view setbacks as opportunities for learning rather than failures. This perspective promotes resilience and long-term success in health and weight management.

Ultimately, the choice between SMART and FAST will depend on personal preferences and the specific context of the goals being set.

THE IMPORTANCE OF COOKING AND MEAL PLANNING

As we so clearly already understand, successful weight management involves more than just "eating better and regular exercise." One critical factor is developing strong cooking and meal planning skills. These skills underpin a healthy lifestyle and ensure that weight loss can be maintained over the long term, providing the tools to make informed and nutritious dietary choices.

The benefits of being adept in cooking and meal planning are numerous. Having control over ingredients cannot be overstated. Research shows that home-cooked meals are generally healthier than restaurant meals. By preparing your own meals, you decide what goes into your dishes, avoiding hidden calories, unhealthy fats, and excessive sugars. When you cook at home, you're more likely to serve reasonable portions, which helps manage daily caloric intake and prevent overeating.

Consistency is another critical benefit of meal planning. Dedicate time each week to plan meals, ensuring you incorporate new recipes for variety. Setting a weekly meal schedule can make grocery shopping easier and help you avoid impulsive eating and ensures that you stick to your dietary goals. Moreover, cooking at home is cost-effective, directing your budget toward high-quality, nutritious ingredients instead of paying for the restaurant markup.

Mastering basic cooking techniques is fundamental to preparing a variety of healthy meals. Grilling, for instance, is an excellent method for cooking lean meats and vegetables without adding extra fats, preserving their natural flavors and nutrients. Steaming is another method that helps retain the vitamins and minerals in vegetables, making them a nutritious addition to any meal. Roasting is perfect for enhancing the taste of vegetables and lean proteins without the need for excessive oils or fats. Sautéing, which requires minimal oil, is a quick and efficient way to prepare a variety of healthy dishes.

KEEPING FOOD TASTY AND ENJOYABLE

Embarking on a weight loss journey doesn't mean you have to surrender your love for food. In fact, perhaps the more important secret to sustainable weight loss lies in finding ways to keep your meals tasty and enjoyable without sacrificing health. Exploring how to enhance your culinary experiences through herbs and spices, utilizing sauces and condiments wisely, and discovering new recipes and adapting old ones will help your food choices remain nutritious and tasty and allow you to savor every moment of your weight loss journey. Embracing diversity, modifying traditional family recipes, and allowing for fun foods maintains a joyful relationship with food.

Exploring a variety of cuisines can introduce you to healthy cooking methods and new flavor profiles that keep meals exciting. For instance, consider the Mediterranean diet, filled with fresh vegetables, whole grains, lean proteins, and healthy fats like olive oil. A dish such as a Mediterranean quinoa salad can be both satisfying and nutritious, combining quinoa, cucumbers, tomatoes, olives, and a simple lemon–olive oil dressing. Another example is Asian stir-fry, where you can utilize an array of colorful vegetables and lean proteins like chicken, shrimp, or tofu, tossed in a light soy or teriyaki sauce for flavor without excess calories.

Revamping family recipes can be a delightful journey, allowing you to keep cherished traditions alive while making them healthier and better align with your goals. Identify opportunities to swap ingredients for healthier versions, like replacing half of the flour in baked goods with whole wheat flour or mashed banana, and use unsweetened applesauce in place of sugar to reduce added sugars. If your family loves lasagna, opt for whole grain or veggie noodles, add layers of spinach or zucchini, and use a reduced-fat cheese blend. Similarly, instead of a heavy creamy casserole, consider a lighter version made with vegetable broth and herbs to elevate flavor while reducing saturated fat. You can also make homemade pizza using whole wheat crust, skipping the processed meats, and loading up on veggies like bell peppers, mushrooms, and fresh basil.

Another tip is to serve smaller portions of higher-calorie ingredients. If a recipe calls for cheese, use less or swap it out for some nutritional yeast, which can add a cheesy flavor with fewer calories. Even better, boost the overall nutrition by adding more vegetables to recipes without compromising taste. Blend spinach into smoothies or incorporate grated zucchini into breads and muffins for added moisture and nutrients.

Maintaining an aspect of fun in your meals is essential for a balanced approach to weight loss. When it comes to "fun foods," indulge in moderation or adapt. If pizza is your guilty pleasure, experiment with a cauliflower crust or make mini pizzas topped with your favorite ingredients. For dessert, freeze bananas blended with a dash of cocoa powder for a creamy, healthy ice cream alternative. By finding healthier adaptations for your favorite treats, you can enjoy them more frequently.

THE BENEFITS OF HERBS, SPICES, AND CITRUS

One of the simplest, yet most impactful, ways to enhance the taste of meals without adding extra calories is through the strategic use of herbs, spices, and citrus. These ingredients are not only flavorful, but they are also brimming with antioxidants, vitamins, and minerals and can enhance the flavor of dishes while imparting various health benefits. For example, turmeric, with its active compound curcumin, is known for its anti-inflammatory properties and can liven up a simple vegetable stir-fry. Cinnamon can help regulate blood sugar levels while adding sweetness to oatmeal without additional sugar or calories. Garlic can improve heart health and infuse rich flavor into a variety of dishes—from roasted vegetables to pasta sauces. Basil and oregano, commonly used in Mediterranean cuisine, are also packed with antioxidants and aromatic compounds.

Citrus fruits such as lemon, lime, orange, and grapefruit enhance flavors with their bright tanginess, balancing rich, fatty foods and adding a refreshing acidity to both savory and sweet dishes. Beyond flavor, citrus fruits are packed with health benefits. They are rich in vitamin C, which supports the immune system, promotes healthy skin, and acts as an antioxidant. Vitamin C also supports iron absorption! So, some lime juice in a chimichurri sauce on a lean steak is an awesome combination! Citrus fruits also provide fiber, improve digestion, and can help lower the risk of heart disease by improving cholesterol levels. So, tossing some orange slices into a salad not only boosts taste but also contributes to overall well-being.

TIPS FOR USING HERBS AND SPICES

Start small. If you're unfamiliar with herbs and spices, begin with familiar options like oregano and garlic and then gradually expand your repertoire. Taste as you go to find balance.

Experiment with blends. Make spice mixes at home. Combine ground cumin, paprika, and chili powder for a homemade taco seasoning that can supercharge fajitas or roasted veggies.

Fresh vs. dried. Fresh herbs typically offer a more potent flavor, but they can be seasonal. Dried herbs are more concentrated, so use about one-third of the amount called for when using dried in place of fresh.

Infuse oils and vinegars. Create your own herb-infused oils and vinegars by steeping garlic, rosemary, or red pepper flakes in olive oil or your favorite vinegar. This adds depth to salad dressings, vegetables, or grain dishes without having to add excess calories.

Layer flavors. Add spices at different cooking stages to deepen flavors. For example, toast cumin seeds before adding them to dishes, or add fresh herbs at the end of cooking for a burst of freshness, or squeeze on some lemon juice to brighten flavors.

SAUCES AND CONDIMENTS

Sauces and condiments can enhance meals and add flavor, but choose wisely, as they can also be sneaky saboteurs with hidden doses of salt, sugar, and fat. High-calorie, high–saturated fat condiments should be used sparingly. Although some sauces can be nutritious, others can quickly add calories if overused.

Nutrient-Dense, Health-Promoting Condiments and Sauces

- **Greek yogurt:** Use as a base for dressings and dips, as it is rich in protein and probiotics. Mix with lemon juice and fresh dill for a delicious tzatziki sauce or stir in fresh herbs for a creamy dressing.

- **Hummus:** Hummus, made from chickpeas, is a fantastic source of fiber and healthy fats. Use as a dip for veggies or spread it on wraps instead of mayonnaise.

- **Mustard:** A zesty addition to sandwiches and dressings, mustard is low in calories and can be a flavorful marinade for meats or veggies. Look for whole grain or Dijon varieties for an extra kick.

- **Salsa:** Fresh, vibrant, and often low in calories, it can jazz up proteins like grilled chicken. Make your own by blending tomatoes, onion, cilantro, lime juice, and jalapeño.

Condiments to Limit

- **Creamy dressings:** Dressings like ranch or blue cheese are often high in fats and sugars. Instead, look for vinaigrettes made with vinegar, olive oil, and mustard or make your own.

- **Ketchup:** Although tangy and flavorful, ketchup can contain added sugars. Limit usage or opt for no-sugar-added varieties. Alternatively, try puréed tomatoes with spices for a fresher taste.

- **Mayonnaise:** Regular mayonnaise is calorie-dense; consider lighter versions or substitutes like mashed avocado or Greek yogurt for creaminess without the extra calories.

TIPS FOR USING SAUCES AND CONDIMENTS

1. Portion control: Use measuring spoons to control serving sizes. Avoid pouring straight from the bottle to keep calorie intake in check.

2. Homemade options: When possible, prepare your own sauces and dressings. This allows you to control the ingredients and customize flavors, making it easier to create nutritious versions of your favorites.

3. Flavor before adding calories: Start by enhancing flavors with spices, herbs, and a squeeze of citrus juice before reaching for a condiment. This develops depth without relying on calorie-dense options for flavor.

EXPLORING NEW RECIPES

Trying new recipes should be an exciting part of your culinary journey, helping you maintain variety in your diet and preventing meal monotony. Explore online resources dedicated to healthy eating where you can search by keywords, like "low-calorie," "high-protein," or "vegan," to discover options that align with your dietary preferences. Invite family or friends to contribute recipes they love or would like to try and make meal prep a more social and enjoyable process. Consider using an organization system that works for you. I like to save the links to recipes I love into a note in my phone organized by meal type (breakfast, lunch, dinner, and snacks) to help with future meal planning.

MANAGING NUTRITION IN THE REAL WORLD

Navigating nutrition amidst the hustle and bustle of everyday life requires intentional and mindful decisions. One practical strategy is batch cooking—spending a few hours on the weekend preparing large quantities of meals like chili, soups, or casseroles, which can then be stored in individual portions for easy grab-and-go meals throughout the week. Cook a big pot of quinoa, roast a large tray of mixed vegetables, and bake several chicken breasts for versatile combinations for lunches and dinners. Chopping vegetables, marinating meats, and preparing grains in advance ensures that nutritious components to create a variety of meals are always on hand. Research consistently shows that individuals who prepare meals at home tend to consume fewer calories, sugar, and fat compared to those who dine out frequently.

EATING ON A BUDGET

Maintaining a healthy diet on a tight budget is feasible with strategic shopping and smart cooking. Buy in bulk when possible, opt for generic brands, and take advantage of sales and discounts. Frozen fruits and vegetables are often more affordable and just as nutritious as fresh. Incorporate inexpensive, nutrient-dense staples like beans, lentils, oats, and canned tuna into your diet. For example, making a large pot of vegetable and bean stew can provide multiple meals over several days at an affordable cost per meal and can be frozen for future use. Cooking at home and minimizing eating out can also significantly reduce food costs.

FEEDING A FAMILY

Ensuring everyone's nutritional needs are met can be easier with a bit of organization and creativity. Involving family members in meal planning and preparation can make the process enjoyable and educational. For example, let kids choose a healthy recipe each week and help them prepare it to encourage positive eating habits. Opting for versatile recipes that meet various food preferences and dietary needs while being nutritionally balanced can simplify meal planning. Preparing a taco bar with assorted fillings like beans, chicken, and vegetables allows everyone to customize their meal. Family meals are linked to healthier eating patterns, better diet quality, and reduced risk of unwanted weight gain.

FAST FOOD, DELIVERY, AND DINING OUT

Eating out doesn't have to result in unhealthy choices if approached mindfully. Look for restaurants that offer grilled, steamed, or baked dishes, and request dressings or sauces on the side. Consider a grilled chicken salad with vinaigrette on the side versus a fried chicken sandwich with ranch. Practice portion control, such as sharing meals or taking half of your dish to go, to help prevent overeating.

TIME MANAGEMENT

Balancing healthy habits with a busy schedule can be challenging, but effective time management techniques can make it easier. One helpful approach is to treat workouts, meal preps, and relaxation times as nonnegotiable appointments in your calendar, like blocking off 30 minutes during your lunch break for a quick walk or yoga session. Focus on high-impact activities that align with your health goals, and let go of less important tasks to help streamline your day. Prioritize preparing a healthy breakfast in advance (when packing lunch the night before) if mornings are typically chaotic. No time to make egg bites? Store-bought is fine! Consider meal prep services that deliver food to your front door! Or kits that provide exactly the right amount of ingredients and an easy-to-follow recipe! Time management strategies are linked to better health outcomes and increased productivity.

STRESS MANAGEMENT

Managing stress helps us maintain both mental and physical health. Incorporating mindfulness practices like yoga, meditation, and deep breathing exercises into your routine can offer big benefits. Spending a few minutes each morning practicing deep breathing techniques can start your day with calm and focus. Engaging in regular physical activities, such as walking, running, or weightlifting, can also significantly reduce stress levels. Walking briskly in nature during your lunch break can clear your mind and boost your mood. Research indicates that mindfulness and meditation can reduce psychological stress and improve overall well-being.

THE IMPACT OF SLEEP

Adequate sleep is pivotal for regulating hormones such as ghrelin and leptin that control hunger and appetite. Maintaining a consistent sleep schedule by going to bed and waking up at the same time every day, even on weekends, can enhance sleep quality. Creating a restful sleep environment with quiet, dark, and cool settings also promotes better sleep. Using blackout curtains and a white noise machine can help achieve optimal conditions. Poor sleep is associated with weight gain, reduced cognitive function, and an increased risk of chronic diseases, emphasizing the importance of prioritizing rest.

WORK FROM HOME VS. OFFICE LIFE

Both remote work and office life present unique challenges and opportunities for maintaining healthy habits. When working from home, establishing a dedicated workspace and sticking to a routine that includes scheduled breaks for movement and meals is essential. Setting a timer to take a 5-minute stretch break every hour can help reduce sedentary time. In an office setting, prioritizing healthy meals and snacks by bringing them from home and incorporating physical activity into your commute or breaks can be beneficial. Taking the stairs instead of the elevator and using lunch breaks for brisk walks are effective strategies. Studies show that breaks for physical activity during work hours can enhance productivity and reduce stress.

Shift Work

Irregular work schedules can disrupt your body's natural rhythms, but implementing specific strategies can help. Creating a sleep-friendly environment with blackout curtains or sleep masks and using white noise machines to block out daytime sounds is crucial for shift workers who sleep during the day. Aligning meals and snacks with your work and sleep schedule to maintain energy levels is also important. Preparing balanced meals and snacks ahead can help avoid unhealthy choices during shifts.

TRAVELING

Maintaining health habits while traveling, whether for work or pleasure, requires a bit of planning and creativity.

For Work

Packing healthy snacks, such as nuts, fruits, and protein bars, can prevent reliance on airport or gas station food. Carrying a reusable water bottle can help you stay hydrated without resorting to sugary drinks. Choosing accommodations with fitness facilities or bringing portable exercise equipment like resistance bands lets you continue your physical activity routine away from home. Utilizing hotel gyms or performing bodyweight workouts in your room are other practical options.

Vacations

Vacations are for relaxing and enjoying, but this doesn't mean abandoning healthy habits. Engaging in physical activities such as walking, hiking, or swimming while on vacation can help maintain your active lifestyle. Exploring your destination on foot or renting bikes provides both exercise and sightseeing opportunities. Indulgence in moderation is also key—enjoy local cuisine but practice portion control and balance indulgent meals with healthier ones. Sharing a rich dessert instead of eating the entire thing yourself allows you to indulge in a balanced way.

SOCIAL EVENTS

Special events often involve tempting food and drink, but a few smart strategies can help you stay on track. Eating a small, balanced meal before an event can prevent overindulgence. At the event, fill your plate with vegetables, lean proteins, and whole grains first and then add smaller portions of treats.

MASTERING YOUR RELATIONSHIP WITH FOOD

The journey to achieving and maintaining a healthy weight is not merely about what we eat; it's also important to understand *why* we eat. To sustain a healthy lifestyle, you need to develop insight into your eating behaviors and identify the emotional and psychological triggers behind them. The GLP-1 medications help tremendously. By promoting a sense of fullness after meals, GLP-1 medications help individuals reduce cravings and the urge to overeat, often leading to more mindful eating behaviors. Consequently, it may become easier to differentiate between real hunger versus emotional urges to eat, ultimately fostering a healthier connection with food.

In real-world applications, many users report reduced snacking or the ability to resist high-calorie trigger foods, enabling them to engage in meal choices more consciously and less compulsively. This shift in behavior not only aids weight loss efforts but also supports sustainable lifestyle changes, allowing the enjoyment food without the burden of emotional eating or guilt. And while helpful, these medicines don't do the work of building new skills or behaviors. It's still on us to learn and practice how to distinguish hunger from cravings, recognize trigger and challenge foods, manage emotional eating, and develop healthier coping mechanisms that aren't food. By honing these skills, you can foster a balanced relationship with food and better navigate the emotional landscapes that often accompany the weight loss journey.

IDENTIFYING HUNGER VS. CRAVINGS

One critical skill in managing your diet and weight is the ability to differentiate between genuine hunger and cravings. Often, we conflate these two terms, which can lead to overeating and poor food choices.

True hunger arises from physiological needs, a signal that the body requires energy and nutrients for optimal functioning. This kind of hunger typically develops gradually and manifests through physical signs such as a rumbling stomach, feelings of emptiness, and a noticeable drop in energy levels. When you are genuinely hungry, your body is open to various food options, and you focus on nourishment rather than specific cravings for particular foods.

In contrast, cravings are often psychological or emotional in nature. They tend to strike suddenly and are closely associated with specific foods, particularly those high in sugar, salt, or fat. Certain foods can trigger pleasure responses in the brain, activating the release of feel-good neurotransmitters like dopamine. Rather than stemming from physical necessity, cravings are typically linked to external cues and emotional states. After a stressful day, you may feel a sudden urge for ice cream or chips, which is more indicative of a craving than true hunger.

GLP-1 medications appear to have the awesome benefit of allowing folks to pause before eating and assess if they are physically hungry or responding to a craving. Taking a moment to reflect can lead to healthier choices. Keeping a food journal can also be beneficial; not only can you document what you eat, but you can also note how you feel at those moments, which can help identify patterns and triggers over time.

EMOTIONAL EATING

Emotional eating occurs when we turn to food for comfort in response to feelings rather than genuine hunger. Common emotional triggers include anxiety, sadness, stress, or even boredom. Science suggests that elevated stress levels and negative emotions can significantly influence eating behavior. People under higher stress experienced more frequent cravings for unhealthy foods as a coping mechanism. Instead of consuming foods out of physical hunger, eating serves as a form of emotional relief, offering a temporary escape from stress. Unfortunately, patterns of emotional eating can contribute to weight gain and further emotional distress, creating a negative feedback loop.

To address emotional eating, it is vital to identify your triggers. Keeping a journal that tracks emotional states leading to eating can provide insight. Recognizing these patterns is often the first step in learning to break them. I challenge you to avoid shaming yourself for your very legitimate feelings. Everyone eats emotionally from time to time—food is comforting and that's okay! Only you can say if the frequency of these events is in need of intervention.

COPING WITHOUT FOOD

Developing healthy coping mechanisms for managing stress and emotions can greatly reduce the reliance on food for comfort and is critical for overcoming emotional eating. Mindfulness meditation increases self-awareness, making it easier to recognize feelings and reduce impulsive eating behaviors. Engaging in physical activity can be another beneficial strategy. Exercise not only helps release endorphins, which boost mood, but also serves as a productive way to channel stress. Activities such as yoga or dancing not only improve mental well-being but also promote mindfulness about your body and how it feels.

Building a support network can significantly contribute to managing emotional responses that may trigger eating. Sharing your feelings with friends or family can provide both relief and insight, creating a sense of accountability. Participating in support groups can offer shared experiences and coping strategies that reinforce motivation. Discovering new hobbies can be an effective avenue for emotional fulfillment and distraction from unhelpful eating habits. Engaging in activities that bring you joy, whether it's painting, gardening, or learning to play a musical instrument, can provide a meaningful and satisfying outlet for emotions.

NAVIGATING FAMILY MATTERS

Any weight loss journey can be positively or negatively influenced by family dynamics. When it comes to addressing these issues within a family setting, approach the topic with sensitivity, understanding, and a proactive mindset.

TALKING TO YOUR CHILDREN ABOUT NUTRITION

One of the most important steps you can take to promote a healthy lifestyle for your family is to educate your children about the principles of good nutrition through modeling and gentle conversations. The key is to make nutrition a positive and fun part of everyday discussions, integrating it into topics like shopping for groceries, cooking meals, and choosing snacks.

Tailor your discussions about nutrition to your child's age and level of understanding. For younger children, focus on simple concepts like identifying foods and understanding basic food groups. For older children and teenagers, discuss more complex topics such as reading nutrition labels, understanding macronutrients and micronutrients, and the importance of balance.

To engage your children in learning about nutrition, try to make the conversation as interactive and fun as possible. Involve your children in meal preparation. Let them wash vegetables, stir ingredients, and even choose recipes. This can be a fun way to teach them about different foods and their nutritional benefits. Children are more likely to adopt healthy eating habits if they see their parents and caregivers doing the same. Make a point to model the behaviors you want your children to demonstrate.

It is also important to recognize and address emotional eating behaviors in children. Help them understand the difference between physical hunger and emotional hunger and what that means for them, and encourage alternative coping strategies like talking about their feelings, engaging in physical activities, or finding creative outlets. Praise and positive reinforcement can go a long way in encouraging healthy habits. Celebrate your child's efforts to make healthier choices and provide positive feedback when they try new foods or help with meal preparation. And it goes without saying: Please avoid shaming or labeling foods or bodies as "good" or "bad."

UNSUPPORTIVE PARTNERS

Dealing with an unsupportive partner can be challenging. The first step is to understand the possible reasons behind their resistance. Some common reasons include:

- Emotional connection: Food often has emotional connections, and changing eating habits can be seen as losing a source of emotional comfort.

- Habit and comfort: Your partner may be accustomed to a particular way of eating and may perceive changes as disrupting their comfort.

- Lack of knowledge: They might not fully understand the importance of dietary changes for improving health and managing weight.

- Perceived criticism: Your partner might feel criticized or judged for their current habits, leading to defensive reactions.

Approach the topic with open, nonconfrontational communication. Use "I" statements to avoid sounding accusatory. For example, say, "I want to eat healthier so I have more energy and can enjoy a better quality of life." Share information and resources about the benefits of healthy eating and the risks of obesity. Sometimes, providing credible sources can help your partner understand the importance of the changes you're making. Identify—together—areas you and your partner can agree on to make small, manageable changes that support your goals. This could be as simple as trying one new healthy recipe a week or substituting water for sugary drinks. Be willing to compromise and show flexibility. Just as with children, leading by example can be powerful. Demonstrate your commitment to healthy eating and an active lifestyle without putting pressure on your partner to immediately follow suit. Over time, they may become more open to joining you in your efforts. If navigating this dynamic proves particularly challenging, consider seeking the help of a professional, like a registered dietitian or a therapist. They can provide guidance and support to help both people align their goals and work together toward better health.

SETTING HEALTHY BOUNDARIES WITH TRIGGERING FRIENDS OR FAMILY MEMBERS

If your family is anything like mine, as a person living with obesity, there are those family members with something to say that is hurtful or unkind—the grandpa who wants to know how much you weigh; the little cousin who makes fun of you in a bathing suit. Somehow it hurts worse when it's family, I know. I've come to accept that the reason people make comments is often a projection of their own internalized biases and struggles.

Setting boundaries with these people is important to maintaining your positive mindset. The first step is to identify what triggers your unhealthy behaviors or emotional eating. Triggers can vary from one person to another and may include:

- Family members who make critical or judgmental comments about your weight or food choices

- People who insist you eat traditional, unhealthy, or high-calorie foods during gatherings

- Family or friends who bring tempting, unhealthy foods into the house or to gatherings or dismiss your efforts to eat healthy

Once you have identified the triggers, communicate your boundaries clearly and assertively. Use "I" statements to express your needs without sounding accusatory. For example, "I appreciate your concern, but I would like to talk about something other than my weight." Setting boundaries requires consistency. It might take multiple conversations before your friends or family begin to respect your limits. Stay firm and consistent in your messages to reinforce your boundaries.

In addition to setting boundaries, focus on creating a supportive home environment. This may include developing a support system of friends or family members who understand and respect your goals. Lean on them for encouragement and accountability.

Sometimes, despite best efforts, family or friends may not respect your boundaries. In such cases, seek external support such as support groups, therapy, or professional counseling. Having an external perspective can provide you with strategies to manage these relationships in a healthy way.

Finally, prioritize self-care in managing relationships with triggering family members. Recognize when you need a break, and give yourself permission to step away from stressful interactions. Practicing self-care ensures you maintain the emotional strength needed to pursue your health goals.

HELPFUL PHRASES FOR DIFFICULT CONVERSATIONS

Try some of these phrases for dealing with commentary from others about your decision to use GLP-1 medications for weight loss.

Polite and Neutral

"Thanks for your concern, but my health decisions are personal."

"I'm happy with the choices I've made for my health, and that's what matters to me."

Firm but Respectful

"I've chosen this, and I don't owe anyone an explanation."

"It's not appropriate to comment on someone else's body or medical choices."

Confident and Empowering

"I'm proud of the steps I've taken to prioritize my health."

"Using GLP-1 medication is no different than managing other conditions with the right treatment—it's just smart health care."

Sassy and Funny

"I'm sorry, I didn't know my health was a group project."

"Are you going to ask Uncle Joe about his Viagra prescription too?"

Setting Boundaries

"It sounds like you have some strong opinions on this, and I do too. I hope you can respect that."

"This isn't up for discussion—let's focus on something else."

"While I'm glad that you're curious and want to learn more, I'd recommend doing your own research or speaking with a health care provider."

CHAPTER 08

SAMPLE NUTRITION PLAN

Buying a meal plan written by someone else might feel like a solution to all your nutrition problems. But, in reality, it's just a stopgap. What if you don't like the foods included? Or don't have access to the ingredients required? Or need to feed a family, not just yourself? Or the time required to prepare the recipes is unrealistic for your schedule? These reasons are why I believe in providing a framework within which to make choices and learn along the way. The first step to making a lifelong nutrition change is taking ownership of the behaviors and efforts required to support it! I know it can be helpful to see an example, so in this chapter, I share some easy-to-prepare, realistic, yet nutritious meal ideas and food lists to get you started.

MEAL PLAN

The following meal plan provides suggestions for seven days' worth of home-cooked meals and snacks for one person on a GLP-1. Each day's meals provide about 120 grams of protein while keeping the total calories to about 1,600. Of course, it's up to you to listen to your body and eat foods that help you feel your best. If these options don't work for you, you are more than welcome to make substitutions!

DAY 1

Breakfast: 1 cup (230 g) fat-free low-sugar vanilla Greek yogurt with ½ cup (70 g) mixed fresh or frozen (thawed) berries, sprinkled with 1 tablespoon (13 g) chia seeds and ¼ cup (31 g) low-sugar granola

Lunch: 6 ounces (170 g) grilled chicken breast with quinoa salad (1 cup, or 185 g; cooked quinoa mixed with chopped veggies of choice, such as tomato and raw zucchini, and a drizzle of olive oil, lemon juice, salt, and pepper to taste)

Dinner: 6 ounces (170 g) baked salmon fillet with 1 medium-size roasted sweet potato and 1 cup (156 g) steamed broccoli; season to taste using a variety of sugar-free sauces or marinades for added flavor

Snack: 1 cup (122 g) carrot sticks or (119 g) cucumber slices with 2 to 4 tablespoons (30 to 60 g) hummus

DAY 2

Breakfast: ½ cup (40 g) oats made with ¾ cup (175 ml) water; once cooked, stir in ½ scoop vanilla protein powder and top with ½ medium-size banana, sliced, and 1 tablespoon (13 g) chia seeds

Lunch: Turkey and avocado wrap made with 1 medium-size whole wheat wrap, 4 ounces (115 g) sliced turkey breast, 1 ounce (28 g) avocado slices, lettuce, and sliced tomato

Dinner: Grilled shrimp skewers made with 8 large shrimp, with 1 cup (185 g) cooked quinoa or 1 cup (140 g) prepared microwavable rice of choice and 1 medium-size grilled zucchini

Snack: ½ cup (115 g) fat-free low-sugar vanilla Greek yogurt with ½ cup (70 g) mixed fresh or frozen (thawed) berries, 1 tablespoon (13 g) chia seeds, and ¼ cup (31 g) low-sugar granola

DAY 3

Breakfast: 2 large eggs, scrambled, with ½ cup (90 g) cooked spinach or (84 g) frozen peppers and onions (thawed) and 1 slice whole grain toast

Lunch: 1 cup (235 ml) canned lentil and vegetable soup with 6 whole grain crackers and 2 mandarin oranges

Dinner: 6 ounces (170 g) grilled chicken breast with 1 cup (162 g) roasted Brussels sprouts and ½ cup (70 g) prepared microwaveable rice of choice

Snack: 1 medium-size apple, sliced, with 1 tablespoon (16 g) nut butter of choice

DAY 4

Breakfast: Green smoothie made with 1 cup (30 g) fresh spinach, ½ medium-size banana, 1 scoop vanilla protein powder, and 1 cup (235 ml) skim milk

Lunch: Tuna salad wraps with lettuce made with 1 can (5 ounces, or 140 g) tuna mixed with 1 tablespoon (16 g) fat-free mayo, ¼ cup (30 g) diced celery, and spices of choice wrapped in lettuce leaves then wrapped in 1 medium-size whole wheat wrap of choice; 2 mandarin oranges

Dinner: 6 ounces (170 g) grilled lean steak with 1 cup (185 g) roasted asparagus and ½ cup (93 g) cooked quinoa

Snack: ½ cup (115 g) fat-free cottage cheese with ½ cup (85 g) pineapple chunks

DAY 5

Breakfast: Chia seed pudding made with ¼ cup (52 g) chia seeds soaked overnight in ½ cup (120 ml) skim milk and topped with ½ cup (70 g) mixed fresh or frozen (thawed) berries and 1 tablespoon (16 g) nut butter of choice

Lunch: 6 ounces (170 g) grilled tofu with 1 cup (225 g) stir-fried vegetables of choice (bell peppers, broccoli, sugar snap peas) in 2 tablespoons (28 ml) light soy sauce and ½ cup (70 g) prepared microwaveable rice of choice; season to taste; consider ginger, garlic, salt, and pepper.

Dinner: 6 ounces (170 g) baked salmon fillet with 1 cup (185 g) cooked quinoa and 1 cup (125 g) steamed green beans

Snack: 2 rice cakes with ¼ avocado and ½ cup (75 g) cherry tomatoes

DAY 6

Breakfast: 3 pancakes (blend ½ cup [115 g] fat-free cottage cheese, ½ cup [40 g] oats, and 2 large eggs, then cook in a skillet like regular pancakes) topped with ½ cup (75 g) fresh blueberries and 1 ounce (about 2 tablespoons [28 g]) nut butter of choice

Lunch: 4 ounces (115 g) deli turkey breast on 2 slices whole grain bread with 1 ounce (28 g) avocado, and as much lettuce, and tomato as you'd like; 2 mandarin oranges

Dinner: 6 ounces (170 g) grilled lean steak with 1 cup (225 g) mixed vegetables (bell peppers, mushrooms, sugar snap peas) in 2 tablespoons (28 ml) light soy sauce served over 1 cup (124 g) cooked cauliflower florets and ½ cup (70 g) prepared microwaveable rice of choice

Snack: ½ cup (115 g) fat-free low-sugar vanilla Greek yogurt with ½ cup (70 g) mixed fresh or frozen (thawed) berries and ¼ cup (31 g) low-sugar granola

DAY 7

Breakfast: 1 slice whole grain toast with ¼ avocado, smashed, 2 large eggs, poached, and 1 medium-size banana

Lunch: ½ can (15.5 ounces, or 440 g) chickpeas, rinsed and drained, in a salad with 1 cup (225 g) mixed vegetables of your choice, like cherry tomatoes, cucumber, red onion, dressed with parsley, 1 tablespoon (15 ml) olive oil, and a squeeze of lemon juice served on 1 cup (20 g) arugula with 6 whole grain crackers; 2 mandarin oranges

Dinner: 6 ounces (170 g) baked turkey meatballs over ½ cup (70 g) cooked whole wheat spaghetti and ¼ cup (63 g) low-sugar marinara sauce, with 1 cup (156 g) steamed broccoli

Snack: ½ cup (115 g) fat-free cottage cheese with ½ cup (22 g) canned sliced peaches

MEAL PLAN SHOPPING LIST

The ingredients here will serve one person all twenty-one unique meals and seven snacks included in the meal plan. Multiply the grocery list to serve a family or buy enough to repeat days and make leftovers or meal prep to stretch this menu to two weeks. And remember, all foods fit the plan, including restaurant meals, processed foods, and convenience items. Not every meal has to be entirely whole foods. You'll also want to use seasonings and add condiments to taste.

Protein (grams listed refer to weight of item)

- Chicken breast, grilled, 12 ounces (340 g)
- Chickpeas, one 15.5-ounce (440 g) can
- Deli turkey breast, sliced, 8 ounces (225 g)
- Protein powder, vanilla, 1 ½ scoops
- Salmon fillet, 12 ounces (340 g)
- Shrimp, large, 8
- Soup, lentil vegetable, 1 can
- Steak, lean, 12 ounces (340 g)
- Tofu, firm, 6 ounces (170 g)
- Tuna, one 5-ounce (140 g) can
- Turkey meatballs, frozen, 6 ounces (170 g)

Eggs and Dairy

- Cottage cheese, fat-free, 1 ½ cups (340 g)
- Greek yogurt, fat-free low-sugar vanilla, 2 cups (460 g)
- Eggs, large, 6
- Milk, skim, 1 ½ cups (355 ml)

Fruits

- Apple, medium-size, 1
- Banana, medium-size, 2
- Blueberries, fresh, ½ cup (75 g)
- Lemons, 2
- Mandarin oranges, 8
- Mixed berries, fresh or frozen, 2 cups (280 g fresh; 300 g frozen)
- Peaches, sliced in juice, ½ cup (122 g)
- Pineapple chunks in juice, ½ cup (85 g)

PRO TIP

Batch cook your proteins, grains, and vegetables at the beginning of the week for easy mixing, matching, and reheating. Not every meal has to be a unique recipe!

Vegetables

- Arugula, 1 cup (20 g)
- Asparagus, 1 cup (134 g)
- Avocado, 3
- Bell peppers, any color, 2
- Broccoli, 3 cups (213 g)
- Brussels sprouts, 1 cup (88 g)
- Carrots, 1 small bag
- Cauliflower, 1 cup (100 g)
- Celery, 1 bunch
- Cucumber, 1
- Garlic, 1 head
- Ginger, small knob
- Green beans, 1 cup (100 g)
- Mushrooms, 1 cup (70 g)
- Onion, red, 1
- Parsley, 1 bunch
- Peppers and onions, frozen, 1 cup (84 g)
- Romaine lettuce, 1 head
- Snap peas, 1 cup (75 g)
- Spinach, one 16-ounce (455 g) bag
- Sweet potato, medium-size, 1
- Tomato, 2
- Tomato, cherry, 1 cup (150 g)
- Zucchini, medium-size, 2

Carbohydrates

- Bread, whole grain, 4 slices
- Crackers, whole grain, 12
- Granola, low-sugar, ¾ cup (92 g)
- Oats, any variety, 1 cup (80 g)
- Quinoa, raw, 2 cups (346 g)
- Rice cakes, 2
- Rice of choice, microwaveable, cooked, 2½ cups (350 g)
- Spaghetti, whole wheat, one 16-ounce (455 g) package
- Wraps, whole wheat, medium-size, 2

Condiments and Other

- Black pepper, ground
- Chia seeds, 7 tablespoons (91 g)
- Hummus
- Marinara, low-sugar, ¼ cup (63 g)
- Mayonnaise, fat-free
- Nut butter of choice

- Olive oil
- Salt
- Sauces and marinades of choice, sugar-free, such as ketchup, barbecue
- Soy sauce, light

EATING WELL FOR WEIGHT LOSS

Assuming your goals are for weight loss and to eat mostly whole foods high in protein and fiber, lower in fat, and moderate in carbohydrates, following are some suggestions by category to keep your meals interesting and on target with your goals. Remember, the overall pattern and balance of your meals (more so than the individual foods) are the keys to success!

PRO TIP

While the foods listed on pages 176–181 and their corresponding protein values are referenced using the USDA database, individual manufacturers and specific foods may include nutrition facts labels that differ, for a variety of reasons. When in doubt, refer to the label on the package of the food you have in hand! Remember, we aren't worried about being exact—close enough is enough!

LEAN PROTEIN FOODS

Essential for muscle repair and growth, lean proteins provide high-quality nutrients without excess fat, supporting metabolism and overall satiety.

Protein	Serving Size, Cooked (as applicable) *grams listed refer to weight of item	Grams Protein
Black beans	4 ounces (115 g)	10 g
Bison	4 ounces (115 g)	29 g
Chicken breast	4 ounces (115 g)	37 g
Chickpeas	4 ounces (115 g)	8 g
Clams	4 ounces (115 g)	29 g
Cod	4 ounces (115 g)	20 g
Cottage cheese, fat-free	½ cup (115 g)	7.5 g
Crab	4 ounces (115 g)	20.5 g
Edamame	4 ounces (115 g)	14 g
Eggs, large	2	12.5 g
Egg whites	4 ounces (115 g)	12.5 g
Flounder	4 ounces (115 g)	22 g
Green peas	4 ounces (115 g)	6 g
Haddock	4 ounces (115 g)	23 g
Lamb, lean and trimmed	4 ounces (115 g)	31 g
Lentils	4 ounces (115 g)	10.5 g
Lobster	4 ounces (115 g)	22 g
Milk, skim	1 cup (235 ml)	8 g

Protein	Serving Size, Cooked (as applicable) *grams listed refer to weight of item	Grams Protein
Octopus	4 ounces (115 g)	34.5 g
Peanut butter powder	2 tablespoons (6 g)	6 g
Pork tenderloin	4 ounces (115 g)	30 g
Pumpkin seeds, dry (kernels)	about ½ cup (52 g)	18 g
Salmon	4 ounces (115 g)	31 g
Scallops	4 ounces (115 g)	28 g
Seitan	4 ounces (115 g)	29 g
Shrimp	4 ounces (115 g)	23.5 g
Snapper	4 ounces (115 g)	30 g
Spirulina, dry	2 tablespoons (14 g)	8 g
Split peas, yellow	4 ounces (115 g)	9.5 g
Swordfish	4 ounces (115 g)	27 g
Tempeh	4 ounces (115 g)	17 g
Tilapia	4 ounces (115 g)	23 g
Tofu, firm	4 ounces (115 g)	20 g
Trout	4 ounces (115 g)	23 g
Tuna, yellowfin	4 ounces (115 g)	32 g
Turkey breast	4 ounces (115 g)	34 g
Venison	4 ounces (115 g)	30 g
Whitefish	4 ounces (115 g)	23 g
Yogurt, fat-free, Greek	½ cup (115 g)	12 g

COMPLEX CARBOHYDRATES

Complex carbs supply sustained energy and are rich in fiber, helping keep blood sugar levels stable and keeping you full while supporting digestive health.

Food	Serving Size	Grams Fiber
Amaranth	½ cup (104 g) cooked	2 g
Barley	½ cup (79 g) cooked	3 g
Black beans	½ cup (86 g) cooked	7.5 g
Buckwheat	½ cup (84 g) cooked	2 g
Bulgur	½ cup (91 g) cooked	4 g
Chickpeas	½ cup (82 g) cooked	6 g
Corn	½ cup (82 g) cooked	2 g
Couscous	½ cup (79 g) cooked	1 g
Farro	½ cup (75 g) cooked	2 g
Green peas	½ cup (80 g) cooked	7 g
Kidney beans	½ cup (90 g) cooked	7 g
Lentils	½ cup (99 g) cooked	8 g
Millet	½ cup (87 g) cooked	1 g
Navy beans	½ cup (91 g) cooked	9.5 g
Popcorn	½ cup (4 g) cooked	1 g
Potatoes	½ cup (113 g) cooked	4 g
Quinoa	½ cup (93 g) cooked	2.5 g
Whole wheat bread	1 slice	3 g
Whole wheat pasta	½ cup (70 g) cooked	3 g
Wild rice	½ cup (83 g) cooked	1.5 g
Rye	½ cup (85 g) cooked	13 g

Food	Serving Size	Grams Fiber
Sorghum	½ cup (96 g) cooked	6 g
Taro	½ cup (66 g) cooked	3 g

VEGETABLES

Packed with vitamins, minerals, and antioxidants, vegetables help reduce inflammation, support immune function, and promote overall health.

Vegetable	Serving Size	Grams Fiber
Artichokes	1 cup (168 g) raw	10 g
Asparagus	1 cup (134 g) raw	3 g
Bell peppers, sliced	1 cup (150 g) raw	3 g
Bok choy, shredded	1 cup (70 g) raw	1 g
Broccoli	1 cup (71 g) raw	2 g
Brussels sprouts	1 cup (88 g) raw	3 g
Cabbage, chopped	1 cup (90 g) raw	2 g
Carrots	1 cup (122 g) raw	3 g
Cauliflower, chopped	1 cup (100 g) raw	2 g
Celery, chopped	1 cup (100 g) raw	2 g
Collard greens, chopped	1 cup (36 g) raw	1 g
Cucumber, sliced	1 cup (119 g) raw	1 g
Eggplant, cubed	1 cup (82 g) raw	2.5 g
Green beans	1 cup (100 g) raw	3 g
Green peas	1 cup (150 g) raw	7 g
Kale, chopped	1 cup (67 g) raw	3 g

continued

Vegetable	Serving Size	Grams Fiber
Leeks, sliced	1 cup (86 g) raw	1.5 g
Mushrooms, sliced	1 cup (70 g) raw	1 g
Okra, chopped	1 cup (100 g) raw	3 g
Radicchio, shredded	1 cup (40 g) raw	0.5 g
Radishes, sliced	1 cup (116 g) raw	2 g
Snow peas	1 cup (63 g) raw	2 g
Spinach	1 cup (30 g) raw	1 g
Swiss chard, chopped	1 cup (36 g) raw	1 g
Tomatoes, chopped	1 cup (180 g) raw	2 g
Zucchini, sliced	1 cup (120 g) raw	1 g

FRUITS

Fruits are rich in flavor, vitamins, fiber, and antioxidants, contributing to heart health, digestion, and reduced risk of chronic diseases.

Fruit	Serving Size	Grams Fiber
Apple, sliced	1 cup (110 g) raw	3 g
Apricot, sliced	1 cup (165 g) raw	3 g
Banana, sliced	1 cup (150 g) raw	4 g
Blackberries	1 cup (145 g) raw	8 g
Blueberries	1 cup (145 g) raw	3.5 g
Cantaloupe, cubed	1 cup (160 g) raw	1 g
Cherries	1 cup (155 g) raw	3 g
Cranberries	1 cup (100 g) raw	4 g
Grapes	1 cup (150 g) raw	1 g

Fruit	Serving Size	Grams Fiber
Kiwi	1 cup (178 g) raw	5 g
Mango, sliced	1 cup (165 g) raw	3 g
Orange, segments	1 cup (225 g) raw	5 g
Papaya, cubed	1 cup (140 g) raw	2 g
Pear, sliced	1 cup (140 g) raw	4 g
Pineapple, cubed	1 cup (165 g) raw	2 g
Plum, sliced	1 cup (165 g) raw	2 g
Raspberries	1 cup (125 g) raw	8 g
Strawberries, whole	1 cup (145 g) raw	3 g
Watermelon, diced	1 cup (150 g) raw	1 g

HEALTHY, UNSATURATED FATS

Although these unsaturated fats are healthy, they should be consumed sparingly. A serving size equals 1 ounce (28 g) or less per meal.

- Avocado
- Nut butter: almond, cashew, peanut
- Nuts: almonds, Brazil, hazelnuts, macadamia, pecans, pine nuts, pistachios, walnuts
- Oils: avocado, canola, olive, safflower, sesame seed, soybean, sunflower seed
- Seeds: chia, hemp, pumpkin, sesame, sunflower
- Soybeans
- Tahini (sesame seed paste)

PROCESSED AND CONVENIENCE FOODS FOR QUICK-AND-EASY MEALS WITH MINIMAL PREP

Let's be honest, trying to eat a diet entirely of whole foods isn't easy to do in the real world. And when nutrition plans are complicated, time-consuming, or high effort, they tend to get left behind. This is where processed and convenience foods are perfectly suited to complement your plan. Knowing you always have something on hand when your best intentions just aren't happening can be a game changer. Here, you will find a list of complex carbohydrates, fruit and vegetables, and proteins that are quick and easy to throw together in a pinch (or on purpose!).

Complex Carbohydrate Foods

- Breads, bagels, English muffins, pita, tortillas, whole grain crackers, wraps
- Canned beans, corn, yams
- Frozen pancakes and waffles
- Frozen quinoa
- High-fiber and/or high-protein cereal
- Hummus
- Instant oatmeal
- Microwavable baked potatoes
- Microwaveable popcorn
- Microwave rice or grain packets

Fruits and Vegetables

- Apples
- Baby carrots
- Bananas
- Canned fruit (in 100 percent juice)
- Canned vegetables (low-sodium or rinsed)
- Cherry tomatoes
- Frozen fruit (for smoothies or yogurt bowls)
- Fruit and vegetable trays (pre-cut and washed)
- Mandarin oranges
- Salad kits
- Salsa, pico de gallo
- Steamer bag vegetable varieties

Protein Foods

- Canadian bacon
- Canned chicken, salmon
- Deli chicken/tuna/egg salads
- Deli turkey or chicken (low-fat)
- Hard-boiled eggs (from the salad bar)
- Lentil soup
- Low-fat dairy: cheese sticks, cottage cheese cups, Greek yogurt cups
- Microwavable edamame pods
- Microwavable egg cups
- Peanut butter powder
- Pre-cooked frozen chicken breast
- Protein bars, powder, shakes
- Rotisserie chicken
- Tuna packets
- Turkey or veggies burgers
- Turkey pepperoni

Mix-and-Match Meal Ideas

Remember, the goal is to include a protein, carbohydrate, and fruit or vegetable in every meal, but that doesn't mean they need to be served separately. If you don't mind your food touching, consider mixing and matching all of your favorites into the following formats:

- Burritos or wraps
- Casseroles
- Fajitas
- Flatbreads
- Omelets
- Pastas
- Rice bowls
- Salads
- Sandwiches
- Soups
- Stir-Fry
- Tacos
- Yogurt bowls

CHAPTER 09

LIVING IN THE MAINTENANCE PHASE

Weight loss is not just about the numbers on a scale; it encompasses changes in lifestyle, habits, and mindset.

Your goal weight may not reveal itself fully until the maintenance phase, as the weight loss itself often involves fluctuations due to various factors, including water retention, muscle gain, and hormonal changes. However, once you transition to maintenance, you begin to see a more stable weight range that reflects your new lifestyle. Maintenance allows you to focus on consistency, reinforcing the habits and skills you've developed during your weight loss, and better understand your body and the weight that feels sustainable for you. Ultimately, you may find that you feel healthier and more energetic at a slightly higher weight than your original goal or feel your best at a lower weight. The maintenance journey is about discovering what works best for your unique body and lifestyle, reinforcing the idea that the number on the scale is just one aspect of a much larger picture of health and well-being.

And—let's be real, weight loss maintenance is hard—arguably, more difficult than the weight loss itself. Let's commit to learning from the past and setting ourselves up for long-term success.

PRACTICAL TIPS FOR SUSTAINABLE MAINTENANCE

Just like the weight loss phase, your GLP-1 medication will work best for maintenance in combination with healthy habits. If we do our part to manage our environment and behaviors, we are more likely to succeed!

Long-Term Behaviors for People Who Maintain Weight Loss (On or Off Meds)

- Participate in strength training at least 2 times per week
- Perform 300 minutes of moderate-intensity cardiovascular activity per week
- Regularly monitor weight (at least weekly)
- Enjoy their "diet" or way of eating, honoring their food preferences and cultures
- Embrace lifestyle flexibility that includes favorite foods
- Enjoy fruits and vegetables (5 to 9 servings per day)
- Prioritize protein as part of balanced meals to stay fuller longer
- Eat most meals at home (limiting fast foods)
- Limit alcohol and sugar-sweetened beverages
- Maintain social supports and long-term provider contact
- Feel as though they have made changes to their identity and are now a "person who eats well" or a "person who exercises"
- Navigate major life changes with grace and without losing sight of weight maintenance goals

Do any of these stand out to you as an opportunity for improvement? **Remember, we want to make sure your habits are in check before we get too stuck on the numbers.**

CHOOSING A GOAL WEIGHT

Measuring success on a weight loss journey isn't as straightforward as counting the pounds lost. If the scale was all that mattered, the most extreme, health-destroying methods would win. But the scale, despite all it may represent in a lifetime of weight struggles, it is simply a tool that most of us have in our homes. Numbers, for better or worse, provide data with which we can make assessments. I get a little annoyed when I hear folks say that "the number on the scale just represents the pull of gravity on your body mass." Actually, that number on the scale reflects the effort and attention I've put into my weight loss journey—thank you very much. It's okay to place some value in it *for yourself*, be proud of it, keep track of it, feel what you need to feel about it, but please do hear me when I say that the number on the scale does not in any way represent your value as a person.

Choosing a goal weight is tricky. It may be less of a choice and more of a feeling or understanding or place of acceptance. The number you have in your mind when you first started your weight loss journey may be different than what is realistic, enjoyable, or sustainable. Having a range in mind though can make your goal feel more real and achievable, so I support the idea of picking a goal and working toward it . . . but how?

Of course, we can start with some basic math using the BMI scale to consider a range within which the "charts" might say we are "healthy." Hopefully, by this point, we know we don't always have to follow these rules and that BMI doesn't always consider body composition. But, for grins and giggles, let's take a look at what a "normal weight" range of a BMI of 22 to 25 might look like depending on your height.

Healthy Weight Range for Height

Height	BMI 22	BMI 25
5'0" (1.52 m)	112 pounds (50.8 kg)	128 pounds (58.1 kg)
5'1" (1.55 m)	117 pounds (53.1 kg)	132 pounds (59.9 kg)
5'2" (1.57 m)	121 pounds (54.9 kg)	136 pounds (61.7 kg)
5'3" (1.60 m)	124 pounds (56.2 kg)	141 pounds (64.0 kg)
5'4" (1.63m)	128 pounds (58.1 kg)	145 pounds (65.8 kg)
5'5" (1.65 m)	132 pounds (59.9 kg)	150 pounds (68.0 kg)
5'6" (1.68 m)	136 pounds (61.7 kg)	155 pounds (70.3 kg)
5'7" (1.70 m)	140 pounds (63.5 kg)	159 pounds (72.1 kg)
5'8" (1.73 m)	145 pounds (65.8 kg)	165 pounds (74.8 kg)

Height	BMI 22	BMI 25
5'9" (1.75 m)	149 pounds (67.6 kg)	169 pounds (76.7 kg)
5'10" (1.78 m)	153 pounds (69.4 kg)	174 pounds (78.9 kg)
5'11" (1.80 m)	158 pounds (71.7 kg)	179 pounds (81.2 kg)
6'0" (1.83 m)	162 pounds (73.5 kg)	184 pounds (83.5 kg)
6'1" (1.85 m)	167 pounds (75.8 kg)	189 pounds (85.7 kg)
6'2" (1.88 m)	171 pounds (77.6 kg)	195 pounds (88.5 kg)

That's quite the range, isn't it? Does the weight you thought you'd be "at goal" fit into these ranges? Yes? Great! No? Still great. Again, there's more to a goal weight than a number. Looking at that chart you might be thinking, *But wait—I thought a BMI of 19 was considered "normal?"* Maybe, if you've been that weight your whole life. Maybe, if you have a very small frame and are very low on muscle. Maybe, if you're extremely tall. But as a person living most of their life with obesity, reaching for a goal weight below a BMI of 22 is unnecessary—and potentially harmful. At a certain point along the weight loss journey, the percent of weight you're losing becomes less and less "excess adipose" (fat) and more muscle and bone. Risking body composition for a lower number on the scale will not improve your long-term health, strength, appearance, or quality of life.

So, we have a number in mind. Let's ask ourselves some questions to check whether this number is going to *work for you.*

1. What weight is actually sustainable to maintain long term with reasonable lifestyle habits without using extreme dieting or restriction? Can you see yourself eating and moving in the same way forever?

2. At what weight do you feel your healthiest? Sleep well? Experience normal digestion? Have good energy? Are in a good mood? Are you continuing to build strength and fitness? Losing too much weight and chronically undereating can feel awful.

3. Where do your previously out-of-bound metabolic labs normalize and chronic health conditions improve? Is your cholesterol normal? A1C? Blood pressure? Liver enzymes?

4. At what weight do you like the way you look? Where do your favorite clothes fit really well? Do you feel more attractive *to you*? If you love your curves, by all means, keep the curves!

5. How much weight loss from your starting weight is realistic based on the medication you're on? Remember, people on Wegovy typically lose about 15 percent from their starting weight; Zepbound is 20 percent, on average. Of course, it's possible to lose more, but plateauing here is common.

I promise I'm not trying to be a buzzkill here, but managing expectations is a skill worth practicing. Coming to terms with the idea that the goal weight you originally chose for yourself may not happen is certainly worth consideration. It's more than okay to change your mind on your goal. Sometimes, we just don't get to choose our goal weight; our maintenance weight choses us. Frustration as you approach maintenance is normal. After six to nine months on a GLP-1 medication, and especially after titrating up to the highest effective dose you tolerate, weight loss slows. The rate at which you lose weight actually needs to slow as you approach your goal. If you're rocketing toward a goal, you may overshoot it at the risk of losing bone and muscle. And if you're not eating enough, you won't feel your best. Remember, improving the quality of your day-to-day life is the ultimate goal.

In maintenance, it's important to focus on nonscale measures of progress and successes to keep your head in a good place. Consider breaking up with the chokehold the number has on your life. Maybe we can find gratitude and self-love exactly wherever our bodies decide to land. Regardless of your exact scenario, I'll share the best advice Dr. Spencer Nadolsky ever gave me when I was struggling with negotiating my maintenance weight: *Fuck the scale.*

Far too often, I see people falling into the trap of chasing "the last 10 pounds (4.5 kg)," and fighting their bodies, their lifestyle, their medicine, and going to more and more extremes to shed more and more weight in search of a specific number on the scale. Sometimes, it's a number they've been in the past. Sometimes, it's an aspirational number their body has never seen. Sometimes, it's a number burned into their consciousness by a doctor or family member or bully from the past. Sometimes, it's an arbitrary number from a chart. Whatever the source, people sacrifice their own best interests in exchange for a number that may never be—and worse, a number that only serves to make maintenance that much more challenging. The risk of rebound weight gain is real. The harder we fight to lose the weight, the harder it is to maintain it. What if, instead of looking for a number, we look for other measures of success. Can we assess body composition? Can we get stronger? Can we improve our diet quality? Can we work toward finding balance between the efforts we put forth to maintain our health and all the other important aspects of our lives that have nothing to do with our weight?

THE SCIENCE OF MAINTENANCE: WHAT WE KNOW

Let's level set with some facts regarding post–weight loss weight regain after non-GLP-1 methods (learning healthy habits, working out, increasing protein intake).

In a typical intensive lifestyle program (without medication) that lasts about six months, includes sixteen or more in-person visits with physicians and dietitians, and nutrition and physical activity prescriptions, folks can expect to lose an average of 5 percent of their body weight, with total weight loss peaking at six months. While 80 percent of participants typically complete these programs (keep showing up to their scheduled visits), only 28 percent of those who complete the program achieve greater than a 10 percent weight loss. Most participants will regain 33 percent of the weight they lost within the first year, and at least 50 percent of participants will return to their original weight within five years.

Then we have bariatric surgery, the gold standard for durable and significant weight loss for folks with the most weight to lose. Folks who have gastric sleeves typically lose about 25 percent of their body weight at two years and keep it off, we think—we are still waiting on the ten-year data. We do know, though, that patients who have had gastric bypass surgery average a 35 percent total body weight loss at two years—amazing! Data shows, though, that even bariatric surgery patients will regain some weight: most average about 25 percent total body weight loss at ten years. Obviously, no method is perfect; 10 to 20 percent of surgical patients cannot lose 20 percent of body weight. For those who can lose more than 30 percent *initially*, 20 to 25 percent of that weight initially lost is usually regained (so if a person lost 100 pounds, or 45.4 kg, they will usually regain 25 pounds, or 11.3 kg) over ten years after surgery. Does that mean the surgery was unsuccessful? No! **I** think this just shows that obesity is truly chronic and multifactorial—it can be managed but not cured.

Why do these folks regain the weight? Well, it's incredibly complicated and probably very individualized, but generally speaking, our environments (obesogenic foods on every corner, socio-economic factors, stress), behaviors (nutrition-related skills, habits, preferences, sleep, exercise), and biology (hello, set point theory and increased hunger after weight loss) do *not* work in favor of keeping the weight off. In other words, our world, our brains, and our body fight back!

So, what do we know about GLP-1s? Let's look at the science . . . The semaglutide research shows that continuing treatment (at the highest dose of 2.4 mg) means continued weight loss maintenance within a few percent.

Body Weight

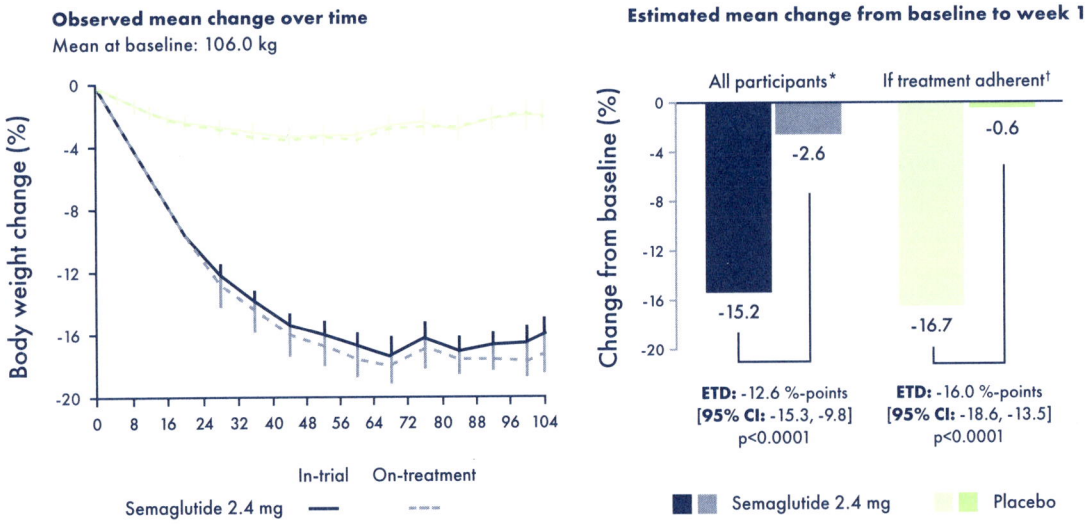

Observed mean change over time
Mean at baseline: 106.0 kg

Estimated mean change from baseline to week 104

*Treatment policy estimated (assesses treatment effect regardless of treatment discontinuation or rescue intervention); Trial product estimated (assess treatment effect if trial product was taken as intended). CI, confidence interval, ETD, estimated treatment difference.

Garvey W.T, et al. Presented at the 39th Annual Meeting of The Obesity Society (TOS) held at ObesityWeek, virtual meeting, November 1-5, 2021.

And discontinuing semaglutide treatment results in pretty obvious weight regain—not for all, but for most, unfortunately.

STEP-1 Trial Extension – Semaglutide 2.4 mg (adapted from Wilding et al., DOM, 2022)

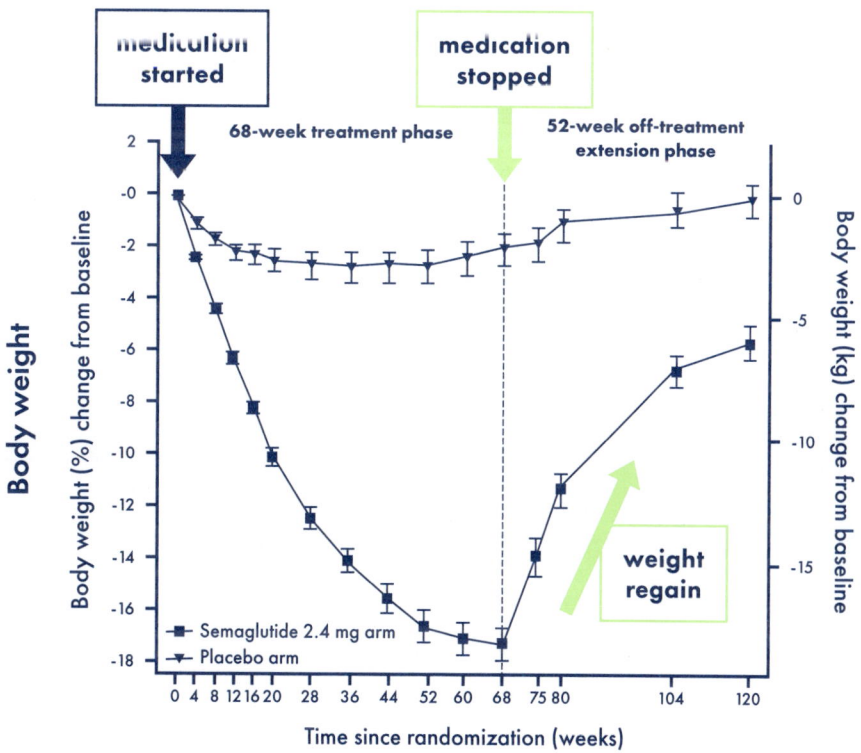

The tirzepatide trials are similar. After three years of continued therapy, weight is generally maintained—of note, not at the lowest weight achieved. I've always found the little bump from 22.5 percent total weight loss to 20.9 percent (while still on 15 mg!) more interesting than the papers tend to address. Do people lose more than 20 percent? Yep! These are averages. But the way averages work, some folks may fall short—sorry.

Percent Change in Body Weight by Week (efficacy estimand)

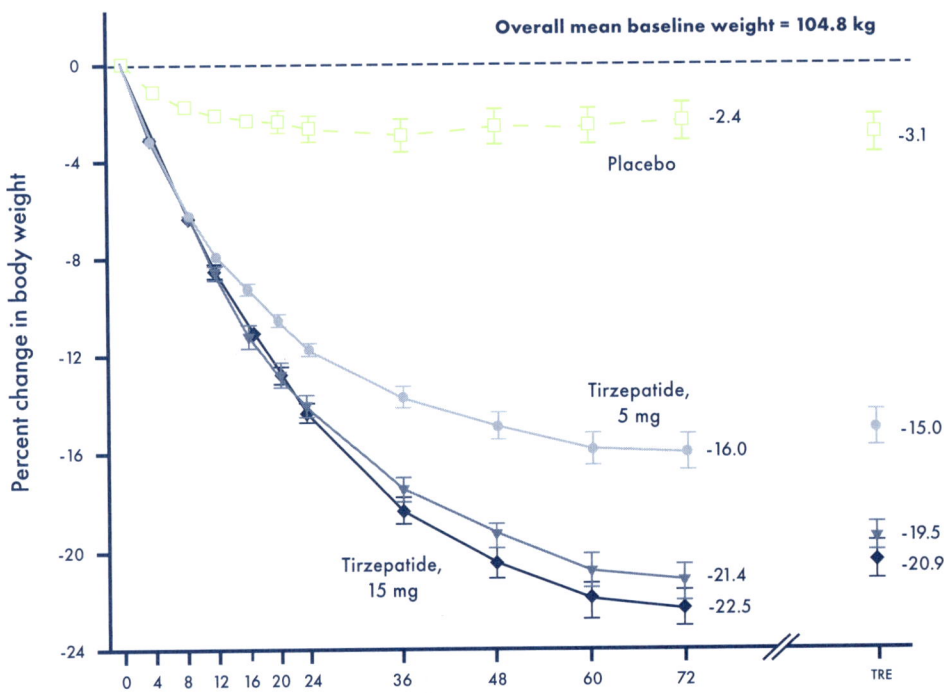

Overall mean baseline weight = 104.8 kg

Placebo: -2.4, -3.1

Tirzepatide, 5 mg: -16.0, -15.0

Tirzepatide, 15 mg: -21.4, -19.5; -22.5, -20.9

Y-axis: Percent change in body weight (0, -4, -8, -12, -16, -20, -24)

X-axis: 0 4 8 12 16 20 24 36 48 60 72 TRE

CASE STUDY

Patient X starts tirzepatide at 200 pounds (90.7 kg), titrates up to 15 mg (like folks do in the clinical trials), and has a typical response to treatment. At the end of 72 weeks, they have lost 22.5 percent of their starting weight (45 pounds, or 20.4 kg) and weigh in at their all-time adult low weight of 155 pounds (70.3 kg)! They buy all new clothes! They celebrate online! They did it!

Check back in with that person at the end of year three, *of course, assuming they continued their 15 mg treatment*, and they probably weigh 158.2 pounds (71.8 kg). This is a win compared to diet and exercise efforts alone. But I imagine this person is frustrated. I imagine this person feels as though they are constantly trying to "get back" to that 155 pounds (70.3 kg). God forbid their original goal was even lower, 145 pounds (65.8 kg) perhaps.

Sound familiar? It's me. I'm Patient X. My lowest weight was 155 pounds (70.3 kg) (well, 152 [70.3 kg] happened for precisely one day). A year later, I'm consistently at 165 pounds (74.8 kg) despite continuing my treatment at the maximum dose. And as a dietitian working with people on these medications, I see this exact scenario play out time and again. The perception of appetite returns, the food noise creeps back in, and the environmental pressures to eat yummy foods you may have been avoiding intentionally start to make more frequent appearances.

Maintenance requires effort despite the meds. And well, that makes sense. Obesity is a chronic disease that is managed, not cured. Had the weight been lost via diet and exercise alone, the magnitude of effort required to prevent a weight regain trend would have been even more apparent. Had the medication been weaned prematurely? Probably also at risk for a gain!

Here's my weight graph . . . working on course correcting currently. But you know *I freaked out* for a while there!

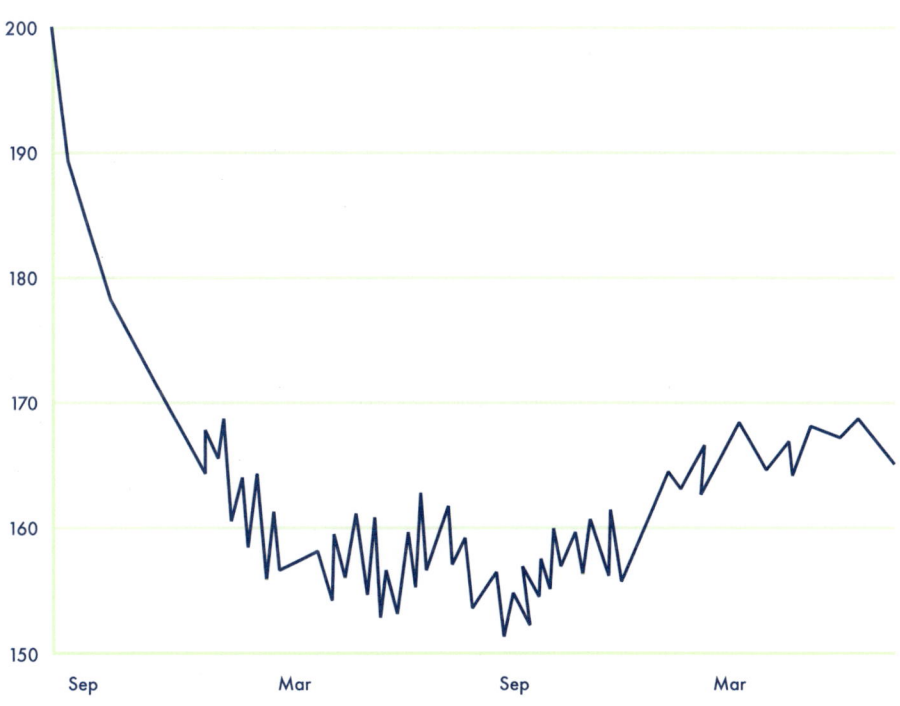

What have I done to mitigate my weight regain? I added back higher-intensity exercise and steady state cardio, reduced the frequency with which I order restaurant meals, and cut back (again) on alcohol that I had let creep back in. When the portion sizes I could physically tolerate were more limited, during the first four to six months of treatment, I could eat less and still lose. But, with all my fitness work and the tolerance I'm building to the medication, I'm a hungry gal again— and I had to be honest with myself about what my life with food needs to look like to maintain my weight!

Some weeks I still "feel" my Zepbound 15 mg doing its thing. Other weeks, I'm starving. So, I have to stay attentive. And I've come to terms with it! It's still, in comparison to the before times, much more doable! Although, if Eli Lilly would like to make me a 20-mg pen, I'd be all in! That original goal of 145 pounds (65.8 kg) is not totally off my radar!

So, as you can imagine, all that said, it is SO INCREDIBLY FRUSTRATING to see GLP-1 programs online "promising" an off-ramp from GLP-1 treatment (looking at you, Noom). We don't have the evidence to say it's possible for most people. Could we try other therapies (old-school obesity meds)? Maybe. Will it work? Maybe. Can we promise? Heck no! I get it though; these major corporate programs are trying to skirt the line between meeting patients with what they need (and offer what the consensus of obesity providers agree on, continued therapy), while simultaneously trying to woo payors (B2B partners, insurance companies) to help control their costs. I also feel badly for folks who hope they can somehow be the unicorn that overcomes all odds and be able to maintain their weight *and* come off therapy. I wish you luck, but it won't be easy.

WHO MIGHT BE ABLE TO COME OFF GLP-1s FOR MAINTENANCE?

I actually have a theory about who can or cannot come off therapy and maintain it. I think there are two types of people who struggle with obesity.

The one type, like me, who has struggled with Food Noise (yes, the capitalized version) and their weight their entire lives. They were overeaters in adolescence and gained weight extremely easily with every life challenge (college, pregnancy, post-partum, new jobs) or even for what seemed like no reason at all. They live their entire lives feeling like unless they are extremely attentive to their nutrition and fitness, they would be extremely obese. We've attempted to lose weight—and probably were successful—a few times but always struggle to maintain, even while continuing the same "healthy habits" developed along the way. We probably, at some point in our lives, had BMIs greater than 40. Those of us like this have that "chronic disease of obesity" that will require chronic therapy. We have those bottomless-pit appetites we never knew could be satisfied until these medicines came along. Maintaining off GLP-1s is likely not going to happen.

The other type does technically qualify for starting GLP-1 therapy with a BMI greater than 30 or greater than 27 with comorbidities. These folks, though, have gained weight recently or situationally. They have lived most of their adult lives at an easily maintained stable healthy-ish weight. Sure, they likely struggled with 20 pounds (9.1 kg) here and there, but never found dieting to be particularly difficult, and if they stuck with it, the weight loss stayed off. They might have gained their excess weight after COVID turned their active lifestyle upside down and now they work from home. Or they experienced a life event that prevented them from eating well or exercising normally—a new relationship with a chef, perhaps. Or maybe they just had a baby and gained more weight than expected. These folks probably have only a little bit of food noise (the lowercase kind). They know what it means to feel full and satisfied. The GLP-1s help them feel good, stick to their nutrition plan, and manage their appetite with less effort, which is fantastic! Good for you seeking a tool to assist. These folks, though, once they've realigned their situations to support a balanced diet and regular activity, probably have the best chance of maintaining their weight long term without medications.

Which type are you?

WHY MAINTAINING WEIGHT LOSS IS HARD

To understand why maintaining weight loss is so challenging, we must delve into the biological mechanisms at play. When you lose weight, your body undergoes numerous physiological changes. Leptin, a hormone that regulates hunger and energy balance, decreases with weight loss. This reduction can lead to increased appetite and reduced energy expenditure as your body tries to return to its previous weight. After significant weight loss, the body becomes more efficient with energy, meaning you burn fewer calories doing the same activities as before. Rapid weight loss often results in the loss of lean muscle mass, which can further slow metabolic

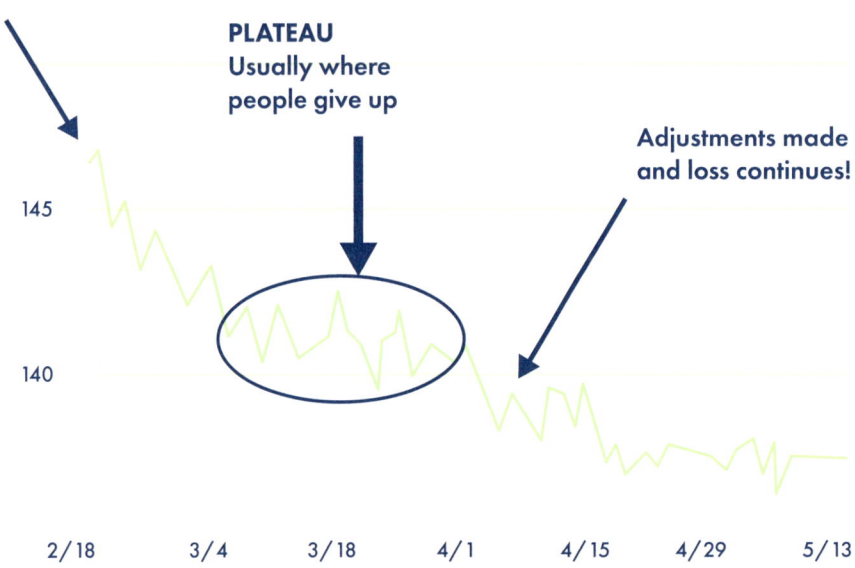

Start of Journey
Initial loss

PLATEAU
Usually where
people give up

Adjustments made
and loss continues!

145

140

2/18   3/4   3/18   4/1   4/15   4/29   5/13

rate (and why strength training and adequate protein are SO important). This metabolic adaptation can make it harder to maintain weight loss without continued vigilance and a willingness to make continued adjustments.

SET POINT THEORY

Set point theory suggests that each individual has a biologically predetermined weight range, the "set point" that their body is genetically and hormonally regulated to maintain. We all know those people who have weighed pretty much the same forever despite periods of more or less activity or changes in diet. Studies have shown that identical twins typically have more similar body weights compared to fraternal twins. This set point is believed to be the weight range where the body (thinks it) operates optimally and so resists changes (weight loss) and "fights back" against variations in diet and physical activity. Unfortunately, this is also why, after significant weight loss, an individual's weight tends to return to its original level over time. When calorie intake decreases, the body compensates by reducing its metabolic rate to conserve energy. Conversely, an increase in caloric intake can lead to heightened metabolic activity to burn excess calories.

Thankfully, there is some evidence that *persistent* lifestyle modifications, such as sustained diet and exercise, can permanently improve one's set point. The dramatic increase in obesity rates globally suggests that environmental factors can override the regulatory systems of our biological set points, for better or worse.

BEYOND THE BIOLOGY

Difficulty maintaining a weight loss goes beyond biology. It is important throughout the weight loss process to also address the psychological aspects of eating behaviors.

1. Incorporating mindful eating practices, such as paying full attention to the experience of eating and recognizing hunger and satiety cues, can prevent overeating and help maintain weight.

2. Social support and environment also influence weight maintenance. Engaging with a supportive community, whether through in-person groups or online forums, can provide encouragement and accountability.

3. Creating an environment that minimizes temptations and promotes healthy choices can make sustainable habits easier to maintain.

4. Regular physical activity is another cornerstone of weight maintenance. The National Weight Control Registry (NWCR), which tracks individuals who have successfully maintained significant weight loss, reveals that consistent exercise is a common denominator among those who keep the weight off.

NONSCALE MEASURES OF SUCCESS

Prioritizing nonscale measures of success can ensure a healthier and holistic approach to weight loss and weight maintenance. Nonscale victories are significant milestones on a weight loss and maintenance journey that go beyond the numbers on a scale. Here's a comprehensive listing of nonscale victories you might practice, experience, and celebrate along your journey:

Physical Changes

- Better sleep quality: Experiencing more restful sleep and waking up refreshed
- Breathing easier: Being able to sleep without interruptions and exercise without shortness of breath
- Clothes fitting better: Clothes that were once tight fit comfortably or become loose
- Easier movement: Simple tasks, like climbing stairs or bending down, become easier to do
- Improved endurance: Being able to walk, run, or exercise for longer periods without fatigue
- Improved posture: Noticing better alignment and posture
- Increased energy: Feeling more energetic throughout the day
- Increased flexibility: Improved flexibility during exercise or daily activities
- Reduced joint pain: Experiencing less pain in joints during movement
- Skin changes: Improvement in skin texture or appearance

Health Improvements

- Better blood sugar control: Improved blood sugar levels, particularly for those with prediabetes or diabetes
- Better breath: Improved breath or oral health due to dietary changes
- Fewer food cravings: Experiencing reduced cravings for unhealthy foods
- Improved cholesterol levels: Seeing positive changes in cholesterol levels
- Improved digestive health: Noticing better digestion and less bloating

- Lower blood pressure: Noticing a reduction in blood pressure readings
- No longer needing medication: Being able to discontinue medications related to metabolic diseases and heart disease
- Reduced risk of chronic diseases: Feeling proactive by reducing the risk of heart disease, diabetes, and so on
- Regular health checkups: Positive results from regular health screenings

Mental and Emotional Wins

- Boosted confidence: Feeling more confident in appearance and overall self-esteem
- Celebrating milestones: Recognizing and celebrating nonscale victories as they come
- Feeling empowered: Taking control of personal health and choices
- Improved body image: Gaining a more positive view of one's body despite scale numbers
- Improved mood: Experiencing a general uplift in mood and reduced feelings of sadness and anxiety
- Increased motivation: Feeling more driven to pursue other goals and challenges
- Less anxiety around food: Developing healthier relationships with food and reducing guilt
- Mindfulness with eating: Practicing mindful eating and enjoying food more
- Resilience: Able to cope with stress more effectively
- Setting and achieving goals: Successfully meeting non-weight-related personal goals

Social and Lifestyle Changes

- Better social experiences: Enjoying social gatherings without anxiety about food choices; feeling more comfortable socializing
- Engaging in activities and challenges: Participating in social activities, like hiking or playing sports, and taking part in fitness or health challenges with friends

- Joining a community: Becoming a member of clubs or groups focused on health and wellness

- Positive influence on others: Inspiring friends or family to adopt healthier habits

- Traveling with more ease: Being able to enjoy travel activities without physical or health limitations

- Trying new activities: Taking up new hobbies or classes that encourage movement

- Self-care: Treating yourself to new clothes, shoes, or workout gear as your size changes

Daily Life Improvements

- Balanced snacks: Creating and enjoying nutritious snacks instead of unhealthy ones

- Enjoyment of cooking: Discovering a passion for cooking healthier meals at home instead of relying on takeout or processed foods

- Experimenting with foods: Trying new healthy recipes and different cuisines

- Grocery shopping changes: Spending more time in the produce section and less in processed foods aisles

- Healthier meal choices: Choosing healthier food options when eating out

- Hydration awareness: Drinking more water and staying hydrated for health

- Portion control: Developing a better understanding of portion sizes

Appreciation of Small Wins

- Completing a challenge: Finishing a fitness class, challenge, or program

- Daily movement goals: Meeting daily step goals or exercise routines

- Game nights or family activities: Playing more active games with family and friends

- Learning about nutrition: Gaining knowledge about nutrition and healthy eating habits

- Progress photos: Taking and comparing progress photos to see visual changes over time

- Self-care routines: Incorporating self-care practices like meditation, pampering, or yoga

- Setting a routine: Establishing a consistent routine for meal planning, exercise, and self-care

- Walking or biking instead of driving: Opting for active forms of commuting

Positively Reflecting on Change

- Creating a support system: Building a network of friends and family for support

- Giving yourself grace: Accepting that progress isn't linear and embracing setbacks

- Journaling: Writing about feelings and experiences related to the journey

- Recognizing triggers: Understanding emotional or environmental triggers related to eating habits

- Redefining success: Redefining what success looks like beyond physical appearance

- Understanding balance: Learning to balance indulgences in moderation

These nonscale victories can be crucial in maintaining motivation and validating the journey to healthier living. Celebrate each achievement, no matter how small, as they all contribute to a holistic approach to health and well-being!

PRO TIP

As corny as it may sound and as awkward as you may feel using them (looking at yourself and speaking them aloud is best), **positive affirmations** can be a powerful tool in reframing out mindset around the number on the scale. Next time you weigh in, give these a try:

"I am more than a number; I am strong, capable, and worthy of love."

"I honor my body by fueling it with nourishing food and movement that feels good."

"Each healthy choice I make brings me closer to a stronger, healthier version of myself."

"Progress is about how I feel, not just what I see."

"I am proud of how far I've come, and I am excited for where I'm going."

"I release self-judgment and welcome self-love into my daily habits."

"I am building a lifestyle that supports my well-being, not just changes my weight."

"I am resilient, and I have the skills to overcome setbacks."

"I am proud of myself for making my health a priority, and I celebrate every effort, not the outcome."

"I trust the process and know that lasting change takes time."

"I love my body for all that it does for me, and I treat it with care and respect."

WEIGHT FLUCTUATIONS

Weight fluctuations while in the maintenance phase after weight loss are normal. While in an active weight loss phase, fluctuations are less noticeable. In our mind, as long as the scale is moving in the right direction, all's good. But in maintenance, when the number on the scale is supposed to be holding still, the usual fluctuations become more apparent. Knowing the common causes of a fluctuation—and what to do about it—can help mitigate the frustration they may bring.

Managing Weight Fluctuations

Once you've identified the common causes of fluctuations and how they impact your weight, you can learn to better manage them. The first step in dealing with a fluctuation is *don't freak out*. A single fluctuation on the scale is not a reason to make any changes to your usual habits or routines. **Consistency in maintenance in your best friend.** Now is not the time to start a new diet or to restrict or compensate or add additional exercise to your routine. Fluctuations, more often than not, average out.

The next step in dealing with fluctuations is to *monitor trends*. Weighing in on a regular basis (whatever works for you) and making a mental note of the ways in which your body responds to what's going on in your life—without judgment—is called "self-monitoring," a key principle in long-term weight maintenance. If you notice a trend, it's time to make some assessments. Are you doing those things that support a healthy weight for you? Are you staying focused on the behaviors and environment that have a positive influence? Are you being honest with yourself? Self-monitoring weight is one thing, but self-monitoring behaviors matters too.

Common Causes of Weight Fluctuations

- Alcohol and caffeine
- Carbohydrates (more or less than usual)
- Digestion (bloating, constipation, diarrhea)
- Exercise and muscle soreness
- Hydration (more or less than usual)
- Illness and injury (inflammation)
- Menstrual cycles
- Sleep changes
- Sodium (more or less than usual)
- Stress

SELF CHECK-IN: KEY NUTRITION AND LIFESTYLE FACTORS THAT SUPPORT HEALTHY WEIGHT MAINTENANCE

- ❑ Acknowledging and appreciating the degree to which your new lifestyle feels sustainable and enjoyable, improves your quality of life, and has become part of your new identity

- ❑ Adhering to a flexible diet in which no foods are totally off limits and fun foods are enjoyed in moderation without resulting in a total detour off plan

- ❑ Developing cooking, food shopping, and label reading skills

- ❑ Doing frequent self-monitoring and course corrections

- ❑ Eating lean proteins with every meal and snack

- ❑ Engaging social supports, like family, friends, health care providers, and communities

- ❑ Getting adequate and restorative sleep and exercise recovery (rest days)

- ❑ Incorporating a variety of fruits, vegetables, and other whole plant foods into meals daily

- ❑ Maintaining confidence in one's ability to overcome barriers

- ❑ Managing stress without neglecting nutrition and fitness goals

- ❑ Minimizing sedentary behaviors like driving, napping, or sitting

- ❑ Performing a consistent strength training routine in which strength continues to build

- ❑ Reducing intake of processed foods high in added sugars

- ❑ Practicing self-compassion in the face of challenges

To maintain your weight loss, you must be committed to maintaining the lifestyle that enabled you to lose the weight—so the elephant in this chapter is: *What about the GLP-1?* It depends. Medication discontinuation is a reality you should be prepared for, as access to GLP-1 medications is never guaranteed. As you've learned, price, supply, and insurance coverage are fickle. But, if we agree that obesity, for you, is a chronic, lifelong, progressive, and relapsing disease with a high likelihood of recurrence, it is more than reasonable to consider that your GLP-1 medication may need to be lifelong.

Available research shows that continuing a GLP-1 medication does maintain weight loss for many years. Some of us were already doing "all the things" with nutrition, fitness, and lifestyle to the best of our abilities and yet, were unable to reach that goal weight until medication was added to the plan. Others, who perhaps gained weight through a short-term life change or series of poor lifestyle habits, may have a better chance of weaning from treatment once these barriers are addressed. In any case, medication decisions should be made in collaboration with a trusted provider and individualized to best serve your unique needs.

When the GLP-1 medication is discontinued, the perception of hunger increases, and a body that has just lost a considerable amount of weight is going to be considerably hungrier. Employing new strategies, like increasing high-volume, lower-calorie foods or perhaps more meticulous food tracking, may be required to maintain long-term weight loss without GLP-1 medication.

LIVING WITH A NEW BODY

A chapter on weight loss maintenance would be incomplete without recognizing the challenges that come with living in what feels like an entirely new body and coming to terms with the way in which your body now moves much differently through the world than it did before. I hope, of course, this is a mostly positive experience, but dealing with the way we see ourselves after weight loss can bring about difficult feelings. Decoupling your own happiness, self-worth, and value from your body size and appearance is key.

What if after all this effort and time you don't actually feel like you look much different? What if the way you look, and feel, now at your goal doesn't line up with your original expectations? Maybe you've lost weight but gained some loose skin and wrinkles. For better or worse, the plastic surgery industry is booming in the GLP-1 era. Maybe your weight loss triggers unwanted commentary from friends and family, or jealousy from a partner, or unwanted attention from strangers. Maybe you're finding that your new access to "thin privilege" highlights the ways in which the "old you" was previously disadvantaged. It can be painful to reflect on the ways in which the world treats you differently. We treat ourselves differently too. We hold ourselves to higher standards or think we don't deserve to be happy or that we are being ungrateful. Whatever the feeling, validate it. It's yours. It's not wrong. And I promise, you're not alone.

APPENDIX: TOOLS

MEDICATION ADMINISTRATION, SIDE EFFECTS, AND WEIGHT TRACKER

Date	Dose	Injection Location	Side Effects	Shot Day Weight	1-Week Weight Loss	Total Weight Loss to Date
1/1/25	2.5 mg	R Stomach	Nausea	200 lbs (90.7 kg)	2.4 lbs (1.1 kg)	2.4 lbs (1.1 kg)
1/7/25	2.5 mg	L Stomach	Constipation	197.6 lbs (89.6 kg)	1.8 lbs (0.8 kg)	4.2 lbs (1.9 kg loss)

30-DAY HABIT AND NUTRITION TRACKER

HIT PROTEIN GOALS: 1.2G/KG+

DAY 1	DAY 2	DAY 3	DAY 4	DAY 5	DAY 6	DAY 7	DAY 8	DAY 9	DAY 10
DAY 11	DAY 12	DAY 13	DAY 14	DAY 15	DAY 16	DAY 17	DAY 18	DAY 19	DAY 20
DAY 21	DAY 22	DAY 23	DAY 24	DAY 25	DAY 26	DAY 27	DAY 28	DAY 29	DAY 30

3+ SERVINGS OF VEGETABLES

DAY 1	DAY 2	DAY 3	DAY 4	DAY 5	DAY 6	DAY 7	DAY 8	DAY 9	DAY 10
DAY 11	DAY 12	DAY 13	DAY 14	DAY 15	DAY 16	DAY 17	DAY 18	DAY 19	DAY 20
DAY 21	DAY 22	DAY 23	DAY 24	DAY 25	DAY 26	DAY 27	DAY 28	DAY 29	DAY 30

64 OZ+ OF WATER

DAY 1	DAY 2	DAY 3	DAY 4	DAY 5	DAY 6	DAY 7	DAY 8	DAY 9	DAY 10
DAY 11	DAY 12	DAY 13	DAY 14	DAY 15	DAY 16	DAY 17	DAY 18	DAY 19	DAY 20
DAY 21	DAY 22	DAY 23	DAY 24	DAY 25	DAY 26	DAY 27	DAY 28	DAY 29	DAY 30

10K STEPS OR STRENGTH TRAINING SESSION

DAY 1	DAY 2	DAY 3	DAY 4	DAY 5	DAY 6	DAY 7	DAY 8	DAY 9	DAY 10
DAY 11	DAY 12	DAY 13	DAY 14	DAY 15	DAY 16	DAY 17	DAY 18	DAY 19	DAY 20
DAY 21	DAY 22	DAY 23	DAY 24	DAY 25	DAY 26	DAY 27	DAY 28	DAY 29	DAY 30

MEAL PLANNING TOOL

	Protein	Carb	Fruit	Veg	Fat (optional)	Flavor	Time
Breakfast							
Lunch							
Dinner							
Snack							

GROCERY LIST TEMPLATE

FRUITS AND VEGETABLES

- ☐ ....
- ☐ ....
- ☐ ....
- ☐ ....
- ☐ ....
- ☐ ....
- ☐ ....
- ☐ ....
- ☐ ....
- ☐ ....
- ☐ ....
- ☐ ....
- ☐ ....

FIBERFUL CARBOHYDRATES

- ☐ ....
- ☐ ....
- ☐ ....
- ☐ ....
- ☐ ....
- ☐ ....
- ☐ ....
- ☐ ....
- ☐ ....
- ☐ ....
- ☐ ....
- ☐ ....
- ☐ ....

OTHER

- ☐ ....
- ☐ ....
- ☐ ....
- ☐ ....
- ☐ ....
- ☐ ....
- ☐ ....
- ☐ ....
- ☐ ....
- ☐ ....
- ☐ ....
- ☐ ....
- ☐ ....
- ☐ ....
- ☐ ....
- ☐ ....
- ☐ ....
- ☐ ....
- ☐ ....
- ☐ ....
- ☐ ....
- ☐ ....

LEAN PROTEINS

- ☐ ....
- ☐ ....
- ☐ ....
- ☐ ....
- ☐ ....
- ☐ ....
- ☐ ....
- ☐ ....
- ☐ ....
- ☐ ....
- ☐ ....

FLAVOR ENHANCERS

- ☐ ....
- ☐ ....
- ☐ ....
- ☐ ....
- ☐ ....
- ☐ ....
- ☐ ....
- ☐ ....
- ☐ ....
- ☐ ....
- ☐ ....

PROS AND CONS OF BEHAVIOR CHANGE ACTIVITY

Activity: Pick a behavior that you would like to change . . .

	PROS	CONS
MAKING THE CHANGE	*Will help you find motivation*	*Will help you consider barriers that will get in the way*
NOT MAKING THE CHANGE	*Will help you see what you might have to give up to make it happen*	*Will help you justify the benefits*

My Personal Current Goals/Example

Increasing to 300 minutes of moderate intensity cardiovascular activity per week

	PROS	CONS
MAKING THE CHANGE	I do love walking! Better chance for maintenance More stamina, healthy heart Tone up my legs Have walking pad already	Requires more time Weather: hot & rainy Family complaining if I'm busier
NOT MAKING THE CHANGE	More time to read/work Can sleep in	Risk for weight regain Feeling sluggish

REFERENCES

Apovian, CM, Aronne, LJ, Bessesen, DH, et al. Pharmacological management of obesity: An endocrine society clinical practice guideline. *The Journal of Clinical Endocrinology & Metabolism.* 2015;100(2):342–362. https://doi.org/10.1210/jc.2014-3415

Astrup, A, Teicholz, N, Magkos, F, et al. Dietary saturated fats and health: Are the U.S. guidelines evidence based?. *Nutrients.* 2021;13(10):3305. doi:10.3390/nu13103305

Butryn, ML, Webb, V, Wadden, TA. Behavioral treatment of obesity. *Psychiatric Clinics of North America.* 2011;34(4):841–859. https://doi.org/10.1016/j.psc.2011.08.006

Donnelly, JE, Blair, SN, Jakicic, JM, et al. American College of Sports Medicine position stand—Appropriate physical activity intervention strategies for weight loss and prevention of weight regain for adults. *Medicine & Science in Sports & Exercise.* 2009;41(2):459–471. doi:10.1249/MSS.0b013e3181949333

Erlandson, M, Ivey, LC, Seikel, K. Update on office-based strategies for the management of obesity. *American Family Physician.* 2016;94(5):361–368. http://www.aafp.org/afp/2016/0901/p361.html

Fertig, AR, Loth, KA, Trofholz, AC, et al. Compared to pre-prepared meals, fully and partly home-cooked meals in diverse families with young children are more likely to include nutritious ingredients. *Journal of the Academy of Nutrition and Dietetics.* 2019;119(5):818–830. doi:10.1016/j.jand.2018.12.006

Ganipisetti, VM, Bollimunta, P. Obesity and Set-Point Theory [Updated 2023 Apr 25]. In: StatPearls [Internet]. Treasure Island (FL): StatPearls Publishing. 2024 Jan. Accessed 2024. https://www.ncbi.nlm.nih.gov/books/NBK592402/

Garvey, WT, Mechanick, JI, Brett, EM, et al. America Association of Clinical Endocrinologists and American College of Endocrinology clinical practice guidelines for comprehensive medical care of patients with obesity. *Endocrine Practice.* 2016; 22(Suppl. 3):1–203. https://pro.aace.com/files/obesity/final-appendix.pdf

Gesteiro, E, García-Carro, A, Aparicio-Ugarriza, R, et al. Eating out of home: Influence on nutrition, health, and policies: A scoping review. *Nutrients.* 2022;14(6):1265. doi:10.3390/nu14061265

Hayashi, D, Edwards, C, Emond, JA, et al. What is food noise? A conceptual model of food cue reactivity. *Nutrients*. 2023; 15(22):4809.https://doi.org/10.3390/nu15224809

Jensen , MD, Ryan, DH, Apovian, CM, et al. 2013 AHA/ACC/TOS guideline for the management of overweight and obesity in adults. *Circulation*. 2014;129 (Suppl. 2):S102–138. http://dx.doi.org/10.1161/01.cir.0000437739.71477.ee

Nauck, MA, D'Alessio DA. Tirzepatide, a dual GIP/GLP-1 receptor co-agonist for the treatment of type 2 diabetes with unmatched effectiveness regrading glycaemic control and body weight reduction. *Cardiovascular Diabetology*. 2022;21(1):169. doi:10.1186/s12933-022-01604-7

Messina, M, Duncan, A, Messina, V, et al. The health effects of soy: A reference guide for health professionals. *Frontiers in Nutrition*. 2022;9:970364. doi:10.3389/fnut.2022.970364

Prescription medications to treat overweight and obesity. National Institute of Diabetes and Digestive and Kidney Diseases. June 2023. Accessed 2024. https://www.niddk.nih.gov/health-information/weight-management/prescription-medications-treat-overweight-obesity

Raynor, HA, Champagne, CM. Position of the Academy of Nutrition and Dietetics: Interventions for the treatment of overweight and obesity in adults. *Journal of the Academy of Nutrition and Dietetics*. 2016;116(1):129–147. http://dx.doi.org/10.1016/j.jand.2015.10.031

Rubino, D, Abrahamsson, N, Davies, M, et al. Effect of continued weekly subcutaneous semaglutide vs placebo on weight loss maintenance in adults with overweight or obesity: The STEP 4 randomized clinical trial. *Journal of the American Medicine Association*. 2021;325(14):1414–1425. doi:10.1001/jama.2021.3224

Sampaio, CVS, Lima, MG, Ladeia, AM. Meditation, health and scientific investigations: review of the literature. *Journal of Religion and Health 56* (2017):411–427. doi:10.1007/s10943-016-0211-1

Simpson, EH, Balsam, PD. The behavioral neuroscience of motivation: An overview of concepts, measures, and translational applications. *Current Topics in Behavioral Neurosciences*. 2016;27:1–12. doi:10.1007/7854_2015_402

Sjøgaard, G, Christensen, JR, Justesen, JB, et al. Exercise is more than medicine: The working Age population's well-being and productivity. *Journal of Sport and Health Science*. 2016;5(2):159–165. doi:10.1016/j.jshs.2016.04.004

Tan, HC, Dampil, OA, Marquez, MM. Efficacy and safety of semaglutide for weight loss in obesity without diabetes: A systematic review and meta-analysis. *Journal of the ASEAN Federation of Endocrine Societies.* 2022;37(2):65–72. doi:10.15605/jafes.037.02.14

US Department of Health and Human Services and US Department of Agriculture. 2020–2025 Dietary Guidelines for Americans. 9th ed. Accessed 2024. https://www.dietaryguidelines.gov/sites/default/files/2020-03/Dietary_Guidelines_for_Americans_2020-2025.pdf

US Preventive Services Task Force recommendation statement: Screening for and management of obesity in adults. *Annals of Internal Medicine.* 2012;157(5):373–378. https://www.acpjournals.org/doi/10.7326/0003-4819-157-5-201209040-00475

Yao, H, Zhang, A, Li, D, Wu, Y, et al. Comparative effectiveness of GLP-1 receptor agonists on glycaemic control, body weight, and lipid profile for type 2 diabetes: Systematic review and network meta-analysis. *British Medical Journal.* 2024;384:e076410. Accessed 2024. doi:10.1136/bmj-2023-076410

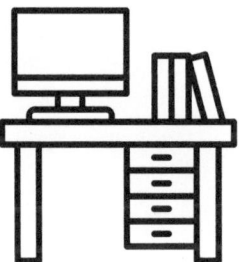

ACKNOWLEDGMENTS

This project has been deeply rewarding and equally challenging, and I am so grateful to everyone who made this crazy idea a reality! As a person who would prefer to do literally anything else than write a paper in school, I knew this would be tough. I am especially grateful to modern technology, specifically voice to text, which allowed me to put my thoughts to text while walking outside in the sun!

In all seriousness, of course, I must first thank my family. To my incredible parents, Victor and Debra, you've raised your difficult daughter into an assertive and authentic advocate for herself and others. Thank you for always having my back, encouraging me to take risks, and knowing that if (somehow, however unlikely) I fail, I will always have somewhere to land. To my husband, Jon, thank you for mostly putting up with my inability to type and talk and listen at the same time. I know it feels like I'm always attached to a screen, and I'm so grateful for your love even when I'm not the most lovable. To my confident and resilient children, Sydney and Colton, you bring so much love and joy to this world and make us all better people. I hope you know that being your mom is the greatest accomplishment of my life. Crap, I'm crying writing this. Okay, moving on . . .

To the incredible team that helped this first-time author learn on the fly and bring this together, thank you for your dedication and hard work. Thank you to my publisher, Quarto, and everyone behind the scenes who worked tirelessly to bring this project to life: Liz Weeks, lead editorial project manager; Anne Re, senior art director; and Emily Austin, book designer and illustrator. To my developmental editor, Mary Cassells, your sharp insights and thoughtful feedback made this book what it is today. I have immense respect for your no-nonsense, time-sensitive approach, and I'm sorry for being such a PIA, truly. You're amazing! To my executive editor, Jill Alexander, thank you for believing in my point of view and giving me confidence to keep at it, even when it got hard. And of course, my technical reviewer, neurodivergent twin, former-professor-turned-bestie, James Gegenheimer; thank you for getting me and contributing your super science powers to this project!

A heartfelt thank-you to my friends and mentors in Obesity Medication Space—most specifically Dr. Spencer Nadolsky—your guidance both professionally and personally has been truly life-changing, and I am forever grateful for you sharing your knowledge and keeping me in check. Corporate health care and the insurance system are harming patients. People with obesity deserve better and more affordable access to medications, compassionate and comprehensive care, more attention, more support, and more trust in this space—and I am proud to help you advocate for that cause.

A special thank-you to my former hospital clinical nutrition manager Hailey Lawyer, you so strongly shaped my early career in dietetics: your confidence in me and support was a welcome gift during a very difficult time in my life, and I'm not sure you ever even knew it! And of course, we must shout out some special dietitian colleagues who influenced my approach, sharpened my skills, and always sent the best texts at the right times: Cristina, James, Allison, Erin, Heidi, and Heather.

And lastly, and most importantly, to my clients, members, patients, audience, community, and online friends: your trust in me as a guide on your nutrition journey is a privilege I don't take lightly. Thank you for inviting me to be a part of your lives and allowing me the opportunity to learn from you. This book is for you, and I hope you find it useful as a source of knowledge, encouragement, and empowerment that serves you well to live your best life, no matter where you are in your journey.

With deepest gratitude,
—Summer Kessel, RD, CSOWM, LDN

ABOUT THE AUTHOR

Summer Kessel, RD, CSOWM, LDN, is a Registered Dietitian Nutrition and a Board Certified Specialist in Obesity and Weight Management with nearly twenty years of health care experience. As a busy mom of two, she is a champion for realistic, individualized, and sustainable nutrition—whatever that means for YOU. In addition to her professional skills, Summer is also a person living with obesity who has lost and maintained more than 140 pounds (63.5 kg)—of course, not without challenges—over the past twenty years. GLP-1 medications changed her life, and she now works to advocate for and educate others on this exciting new world of weight loss and nutrition!

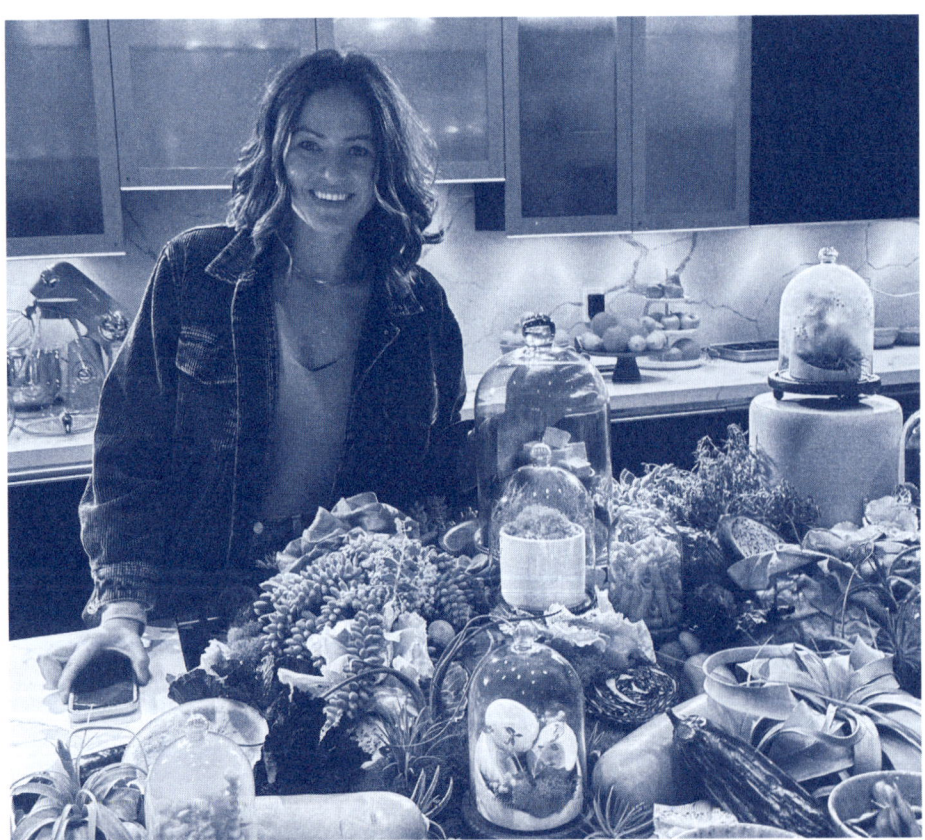

INDEX